中国本科医学教育标准——
临床医学专业

（2022 版）

教育部临床医学专业认证工作委员会

北京大学医学出版社

ZHONGGUO BENKE YIXUE JIAOYU BIAOZHUN—
LINCHUANG YIXUE ZHUANYE（2022 BAN）

图书在版编目（CIP）数据

中国本科医学教育标准—临床医学专业：2022版/
教育部临床医学专业认证工作委员会编．—北京：北京
大学医学出版社，2023.3（2024.3重印）
ISBN 978-7-5659-2855-0

Ⅰ．①中…　Ⅱ．①教…　Ⅲ．①临床医学－本科－医学
教育－标准－中国　Ⅳ．①R-4

中国国家版本馆CIP数据核字（2023）第027820号

中国本科医学教育标准—临床医学专业（2022版）

编： 教育部临床医学专业认证工作委员会
出版发行： 北京大学医学出版社
地　　址： （100191）北京市海淀区学院路38号　北京大学医学部院内
电　　话： 发行部 010-82802230；图书邮购 010-82802495
网　　址： http://www.pumpress.com.cn
E - m a i l： booksale@bjmu.edu.cn
印　　刷： 北京瑞达方舟印务有限公司
经　　销： 新华书店
责任编辑： 赵　欣　孙敬怡　韩忠刚　　**责任校对：** 靳新强　　**责任印制：** 李　啸
开　　本： 880 mm×1230 mm　1/32　**印张：** 5　**字数：** 75千字
版　　次： 2023 年 3 月第 1 版　2024 年 3 月第 2 次印刷
书　　号： ISBN 978-7-5659-2855-0
定　　价： 20.00元

前　言

　　医学教育承载着培养医药卫生人才的使命，与全民健康息息相关。自 2008 年教育部和原卫生部颁布《本科医学教育标准—临床医学专业（试行）》之后，我国逐步开展了本科临床医学专业认证工作，成立了教育部临床医学专业认证工作委员会（以下简称"工作委员会"），颁布了《临床医学专业认证指南（试行）》，初步建立了中国临床医学专业认证制度。2016 年，工作委员会正式发布《中国本科医学教育标准—临床医学专业（2016 版）》，并将其作为新一轮认证的依据。

　　2020 年 6 月，工作委员会正式获得世界医学教育联合会（World Federation for Medical Education，WFME）医学教育认证机构认定，标志着我国医学教育标准和认证体系已实现国际实质等效，医学教育认证质量得到了国际认可。截至 2021 年底，工作委员会完成了我国高等医学院校的本科临床医学专业首轮认证。

　　为保证医学教育标准的与时俱进，更好地推进新一轮本科临床医学专业认证实践，工作委员会总结我国本科临床医学专业认证的有益经验，及时引进医学教育最新理念，于 2021 年启动对 2016 版标准的修订工作，形成《中国本科医学教育标准—临床医学专业（2022 版）》。

2022 版标准仍由临床医学专业本科毕业生应达到的基本要求和临床医学专业本科医学教育办学标准两部分组成。在临床医学专业本科医学教育办学标准部分，仍分为基本标准（basic standards，B）和发展标准（quality development standards，Q）。基本标准为所有举办临床医学专业本科教育的院校都必须达到的标准，用"必须"来表达。发展标准为国际所倡导的本科临床医学教育高标准，体现了医学教育发展的方向，用"应当"来表达，达成情况因各医学院校的不同发展阶段、资源状况和教育政策而有所不同。与 2016 版标准相比，2022 版办学标准部分的主领域仍为 10 个，亚领域仍为 40 个；条目由原来的 113 条基本标准和 80 条发展标准调整为 117 条基本标准和 76 条发展标准。同时，为增加可读性，对注释内容增加了数字索引（annotations，A），共 86 条。

本标准适用于临床医学专业本科教育阶段，是临床医学专业认证的依据。本科医学教育是医学教育连续体中的第一阶段，其根本任务是培养完成医学基本训练，具有初步临床能力、终身学习能力和良好职业精神与素养的医学毕业生。本科医学教育为学生接受毕业后教育和在各类卫生保健机构执业奠定必要的基础。医学本科毕业生胜任临床工作的专业能力需要在毕业后医学教育、继续职业发展和持续医疗实践中逐渐形成与提高。

本标准反映医学教育的国际趋势、国内现状和社会期待，是制订教育计划和规范教学管理的依据。各医学院校应在标准的指导下，确立自身的办学定位，制订专业的培养目标和课程计划，建立教育评价体系和质量保障机制。

本标准承认不同地区和学校之间的差异，尊重学校办学自主权。在遵循医学教育基本规律的前提下，除必要的要求外，不对课程计划提出过多具体的、强制性的规定，为各校的发展及办学留下充分的空间。应该着重强调的是，本标准贯彻党的教育方针，坚持立德树人，致力于指导我国临床医学专业办学实践，提高医学人才培养质量。

目　录

临床医学专业本科毕业生应达到的基本要求

中国临床医学专业本科毕业生应树立正确的世界观、人生观、价值观，热爱祖国，忠于人民，遵纪守法，愿为祖国医药卫生与健康事业的发展和人类身心健康奋斗终生。

中国临床医学专业本科毕业生应达到的基本要求分为四个领域：科学和学术、临床能力、健康与社会、职业精神与素养。每所院校可根据实际情况，对毕业生的预期结果提出更具体的要求。

医学教育是一个包括院校教育、毕业后教育和继续职业发展的连续过程。经过院校教育的本科毕业生具备了相应的从业基础，但尚不具备丰富的临床经验，这就要求他们在日新月异的医学进步环境中保持其医学业务水平的持续更新。毕业生在校期间获得的教育培训以及掌握的科学方法将为他们终身学习与发展提供支撑。

1 科学和学术领域

1.1 具备自然科学、人文社会科学、医学等学科的基础知识，掌握科学方法，并能用于指导未来的学习和医学实践。

1.2 能够应用医学等科学知识处理个体、群体和卫生系统中与医学或者健康相关的问题。

1.3 能够理解和描述生命各阶段疾病的预防和疾病的病因、发病机制、病程、临床表现、诊断、治疗、转归、预后及康复。

1.4 能够掌握中医药学的基本特点和诊疗基本原则。

1.5 能够获取、甄别、理解并应用医学等科学文献中的证据。

1.6 能够应用常用的科学方法，提出相应的科学问题并进行探讨。

2 临床能力领域

2.1 具有良好的交流沟通能力，能够与患者及其家属或监护人、同行和其他卫生专业人员等进行有效的交流。

2.2 能够全面、系统、正确地采集病史。

2.3 能够系统、规范地进行体格检查及精神状态评价，规范地书写病历。

2.4 能够依据病史和体格检查中的发现，形成初步判断，并进行鉴别诊断，提出合理的治疗原则。

2.5 能够根据患者的病情、安全和成本效益等因素，选择适宜的临床检查方法并说明其合理性，对检查结果能做出判断和解释。

2.6 能够选择并安全地实施常用的临床基本操作。

2.7 能够根据不断获取的证据做出临床判断和决策，在上级医师指导下确定进一步的诊疗方案并说明其合理性。

2.8 能够了解患者的问题、意见、关注点和偏好，使患者及其家属或监护人充分理解病情；就诊疗方案的风险和益处同患者及其家属或监护人进行沟通，并共同制订诊疗计划（医患共同决策）。

2.9 能够及时向患者及其家属或监护人提供相关信息，使他们在充分知情的前提下选择诊疗方案。

2.10 能够将疾病预防、早期发现、卫生保健和慢性疾病管理等知识和理念应用于临床实践。

2.11 能够依据客观证据，提出安全、有效、经济的治疗方案。

2.12 能够发现并评价病情的变化及严重程度，对需要紧急处理的患者进行可能的急救处理。

2.13 能够掌握临终患者的治疗原则，与患者家属或监护人沟通。用对症、心理支持等姑息治疗的方法达到人道主义的目的，提高患者的死亡质量。

2.14　能够在临床信息系统中有效地检索、解读和记录信息。

3　健康与社会领域

3.1　具有保护并促进个体和人群健康的责任意识。

3.2　能够了解影响人群健康、疾病诊断和有效治疗的因素，包括健康公平性、文化和社会价值观的多样性，以及社会经济、心理状态和自然环境等因素。

3.3　能够在不同情境下以不同的角色进行有效沟通，如医生、健康倡导者、研究者等。

3.4　能够解释和评估人群的健康检查和预防措施，包括人群健康状况的监测、患者随访、用药、康复治疗及其他方面的指导等。

3.5　能够了解医院医疗质量保障和医疗安全管理体系，明确自己的业务能力与权限，重视患者安全，及时识别对患者不利的危险因素。

3.6　能够了解我国医疗卫生系统的结构和功能，以及各组成部门的职能和相互关系，理解合理分配有限资源的原则，以满足个人、群体和国家对健康的需求。

3.7　能够了解全球健康问题以及健康和疾病的影响因素。

4　职业精神与素养领域

4.1　能够根据《中国医师道德准则》，为所有患者提供人道主义的医疗服务。

4.2　能够了解医疗卫生领域职业精神的内涵，在工作中养成同理心、尊重患者和提供优质服务等行为，形成真诚、正直、团队合作和领导力等素养。

4.3　能够掌握医学伦理学的主要原理，并将其应用于医疗服务中。能够与患者及其家属或监护人、同行和其他卫生专业人员等有效地沟通伦理问题。

4.4　能够了解影响医生健康的因素，如疲劳、压力和交叉感染等，并注意在医疗服务中有意识地控制这些因素，同时知晓自身健康对患者可能构成的风险。

4.5　能够了解并遵守医疗行业的基本法律法规和职业道德。

4.6　能够意识到自己专业知识的局限性，尊重其他卫生从业人员，并注重相互合作和学习。

4.7　树立自主学习、终身学习的观念，认识到持续自我完善的重要性，不断追求卓越。

临床医学专业本科医学教育办学标准

1 宗旨与结果

1.1 宗旨

基本标准：

医学院校必须：

- 具有明确的办学宗旨，并让全校师生员工、医疗卫生机构等利益相关方知晓。（B 1.1.1）
- 在宗旨中阐述医学生培养的总体目标及实现策略，确保医学生在毕业时能够达到临床医学专业本科毕业生的基本要求。（B 1.1.2）
- 确保宗旨在相关法律框架内满足医疗服务体系和公众健康的需求，同时兼顾其他方面的社会责任。（B 1.1.3）

发展标准：

医学院校应当：

- 在宗旨中包括：
  - 医学研究的目标定位。（Q 1.1.1）
  - 对大健康理念和全球卫生观念的要求。（Q 1.1.2）

【注释】

- *宗旨*阐述医学教育办学的总体框架，包括办学定位、办学理念、人才培养目标等。宗旨的制定应与学校的资源、管理相适应，同时考虑地方与国家、区域与全球对医学的期望和发展的需要，并体现学校历史文化积淀和发展愿景。办学定位应体现学校的办学类型、办学层次、服务面向、发展目标等；办学理念应体现学校人才培养的教育思想和观念。（A 1.1.1）

- *医学院校*是指提供本科临床医学专业教育的教育机构，可以是独立建制院校，也可以是综合性大学的一部分。医学院校还应包括附属医院及其他临床教学基地。医学院校不仅提供本科医学教育、开展研究、提供医疗服务，还可为医学教育的其他阶段或其他卫生相关行业提供教育方案和实施保障。（A 1.1.2）

- *满足公众健康的需求*是指与当地卫生及其相关部门进行沟通，通过调整课程计划来表明对当地公众健康问题的了解和关注。（A 1.1.3）

- *社会责任*是指有意愿和能力通过提高医疗服务、医学教育及医学研究能力来满足社会、患者、卫生及其相关部门的需要，促进国家和全球医学事业的发展。社会责任应以尊重医学院校办学自主权为基础。超出医学院校权限的问题，尤其是医疗卫生相关问题，可以通过表明态度、分析因果关系以及提出相应建议等方式展现其社会责任。（A 1.1.4）

- *医学研究包含生物与基础医学、临床医学、公共卫生与预防医学以及其他与医学相关的科学研究。*（A 1.1.5）

- *全球卫生观念是指对全球范围内不同区域主要健康问题的认知，包括对全球共同面临的健康问题和对因种族差异、地域差别、贫富不均等所引起的不平等与不公平的健康问题的认识，以及为应对这些健康问题的挑战而需要开展的跨学科、跨部门、多行为体参与的全球卫生治理的认识。*（A 1.1.6）

1.2 宗旨制定过程的参与

基本标准：

医学院校必须：

- 保证校内主要利益相关方参与宗旨的制定。（B 1.2.1）

发展标准：

医学院校应当：

- 具有校外利益相关方参与宗旨制定的机制，并有效实施。（Q 1.2.1）

【注释】

- *校内主要利益相关方包括教师、学生、校 / 院领导和行政管理人员。*（A 1.2.1）
- *校外利益相关方包括相关政府机构和主管部门、用人单位、社区和公众代表、学术和管理部门、专业学术团体、医学科研组织和毕业后教育机构的代表等。*（A 1.2.2）

1.3　院校自主权和学术自由

基本标准：

医学院校必须：

- 拥有在符合相关法律、法规的前提下，制定和实施各项政策的自主权，尤其是在以下方面：
  - 课程计划的制定。（B 1.3.1）
  - 课程计划实施所需资源的配置与使用。（B 1.3.2）
- 得到大学自然科学、人文社会科学等学科对医学教育的学术支持。（B 1.3.3）
- 保证教师和学生拥有学术自由。（B 1.3.4）

发展标准：

医学院校应当：

- 加强人文社会学科、自然学科与医学学科间的融合。（Q 1.3.1）

【注释】

- *院校自主权*是指医学院校相对独立于政府或其他相关部门（区域及地方行政部门、私人合作方、行业协会、联盟和与临床医学专业相关的其他利益相关组织等），对招生、课程计划、评价考核、教师聘任及待遇、科研和资源配置等关键问题有自主决策权。院校自主权应以遵守国家法律法规和遵循医学教育基本发展规律为前提。（A 1.3.1）

- *学术自由*应以遵守国家法律法规为前提。（A 1.3.2）

1.4 教育结果

基本标准：

医学院校必须：

- 明确规定医学生毕业时在科学和学术、临床能力、健康与社会、职业精神与素养四大领域的基本要求，阐明与办学宗旨目标相适应

的毕业生教育结果。（B 1.4.1）

- 阐明学生在与同伴、教师、医疗服务领域其他从业者、患者及其家属或监护人相处时应有的恰当的行为方式。（B 1.4.2）

发展标准：

医学院校应当：

- 明确建立院校教育结果和毕业后教育之间的关系。（Q 1.4.1）
- 明确学生参与医学相关研究的要求以及期望的结果。（Q 1.4.2）
- 明确学生对于大健康与全球卫生状况认识水平的要求。（Q 1.4.3）

【注释】

- *教育结果*可以通过相应手段进行测量和评价，如学业考核、学生综合评价、学生发展和毕业生调查、就业与职业发展状况分析等。学业考核包括课程考核、毕业考核、医学院校临床医学专业（本科）水平测试、国家临床执业医师资格考试等。（A 1.4.1）

2　课程计划

2.1　课程计划的制定与实施

基本标准：

医学院校必须：

- 依据医药卫生与健康事业的需要、医学科学的进步和医学模式的转变，制定与本校宗旨、目标、教育结果相适应的课程计划。（B 2.1.1）
- 在课程计划中体现加强基础、培养能力、注重素质和发展个性的原则。（B 2.1.2）
- 明确课程模式。（B 2.1.3）
- 阐明根据不同的课程目标、内容和教学对象所采用的适宜教学方法。（B 2.1.4）
- 确保课程计划和教学方法能够激发、培养和支持学生自主学习。（B 2.1.5）
- 以平等的原则实施课程计划。（B 2.1.6）

发展标准：

医学院校应当：

- 对学生自主学习和终身学习能力的培养有科学、系统的设计与实施。（Q 2.1.1）
- 在课程计划中体现科学发展新趋势。（Q 2.1.2）

【注释】

- *课程计划包括培养目标、预期结果、课程模式、课程设置（课程结构、组成、学分和时间分配）和考核原则等。课程计划应有与之相匹配的课程教学大纲。课程教学大纲涵盖课程教学目标、教学内容、教学方法、学习资源、考核要求等内容，各部分应相互协调，并与培养目标相适应。*（A 2.1.1）

- *课程模式可以是基于学科的模式，也可以是各种整合模式。*（A 2.1.2）

- *教学方法含教与学两个方面，包括课堂讲授、小组讨论、基于问题或案例的学习、同伴学习、实验教学、临床示教、床旁教学、临床技能训练、情景教学、模拟/虚拟教学、线上线下混合教学等。*（A 2.1.3）

- *自主学习指学习者自我驱动，判断自身的学习需求，制定适合自己的学习目标，辨别与整合相关的学习内容与资源，选择适当的学习方法与策略，监控自身的学习过程，评价自身的学习效果，并不断调节自身的学习行为。*（A 2.1.4）

- *平等的原则是指学校在教学实施过程中遵守

公平性和多样化的原则。在制定教学管理、学生评价等方面的规章制度时充分考虑学生的性别、民族、宗教、文化、社会背景等。（A 2.1.5）

- *课程计划和教学方法需要以现代学习理论为基础。*（A 2.1.6）

2.2　科学方法教育

基本标准：

医学院校必须：

- 在整个课程计划中包括：
  - 科学方法原理，强调分析和解决问题的能力、批判性思维的培养。（B 2.2.1）
  - 医学研究方法的训练。（B 2.2.2）
  - 循证医学教育。（B 2.2.3）

发展标准：

医学院校应当：

- 鼓励和支持学生参与科学研究，并将学生科研训练纳入课程计划。（Q 2.2.1）
- 将原创的或前沿的研究纳入教学过程中。（Q 2.2.2）
- 将科学方法原理、医学研究方法和创新意识的教育贯穿人才培养的全过程。（Q 2.2.3）

【注释】

- *科学方法教育指教学过程中对科学方法和科学意识的培养。*（A 2.2.1）

2.3 人文社会科学和自然科学课程

基本标准：

医学院校必须：

- 在整个课程计划中覆盖下列领域的内容：
  - 人文社会科学，特别强调思想道德修养、医学伦理、卫生法律法规等内容。（B 2.3.1）
  - 自然科学。（B 2.3.2）

发展标准：

医学院校应当：

- 将人文社会科学融入医学专业教学中，重视职业精神与素养的培养。调整并优化课程计划中人文社会科学的内容和权重，以适应：
  - 科学技术和临床医学发展。（Q 2.3.1）
  - 社会和医疗卫生体系当前和未来的需求。（Q 2.3.2）
  - 不断变化的人口和文化环境的需要。（Q 2.3.3）

【注释】

- 人文社会科学包括医学史、医学伦理、卫生

法、医学心理、医学社会、卫生事业管理等
方面的内容，其内容涵盖的广度和深度取决
于医学院校教育目标的要求。鼓励将人文社
会科学知识内容进行整合并融入专业课程教
学。（A 2.3.1）

- *自然科学包括数学、物理、化学等内容。*
  （A 2.3.2）

2.4　生物与基础医学课程

基本标准：

医学院校必须：

- 在课程计划中开设生物与基础医学课程，使
  学生全面了解医学科学知识，掌握基本概念和
  方法，并了解其在临床中的应用。（B 2.4.1）

发展标准：

医学院校应当：

- 根据科学技术和医学发展以及社会对卫生
  保健服务的需求调整生物与基础医学课程。
  （Q 2.4.1）

【注释】

- *生物与基础医学课程包括人体解剖学（含系*
  统解剖与局部解剖）、组织学与胚胎学、细
  胞生物学、医学遗传学、生物化学与分子

生物学、生理学、病原生物学、医学免疫学、病理学、药理学、病理生理学等核心课程或内容；以及与医学学科发展相关的拓展课程或内容，如神经生物学。以上课程或内容也可以整合的形式呈现。核心课程或内容应列为必修，拓展课程或内容依培养目标和院校资源情况自主设置并可列为必修或选修。（A 2.4.1）

2.5 公共卫生与预防医学课程

基本标准：

医学院校必须：

- 安排公共卫生与预防医学相关内容，培养学生的预防战略和公共卫生意识，使其掌握健康教育和健康促进的知识与技能，并能应用于临床实践。（B 2.5.1）

发展标准：

医学院校应当：

- 将公共卫生与预防医学相关内容融入医学教育全过程。（Q 2.5.1）
- 使学生了解全球卫生的状况，具有全球卫生意识。（Q 2.5.2）

【注释】

- 公共卫生与预防医学相关内容包括医学统计学、流行病学、妇幼与儿少卫生学、社会医学、环境卫生学、营养与食品卫生学、劳动卫生与职业病学、全球卫生、健康教育与健康促进等。（A 2.5.1）

2.6 临床医学课程

基本标准：

医学院校必须：

- 在课程计划中明确并涵盖临床学科内容，确保学生获得全面的临床医学知识、临床能力、职业精神与素养，在毕业后能够承担相应的临床工作。（B 2.6.1）
- 在临床环境中安排临床医学课程，确保学生有足够的时间接触患者，并做出合理的教学安排。（B 2.6.2）
- 保证理论授课和临床见习紧密结合。（B 2.6.3）
- 确保学生在本校附属医院及与本校签有书面协议、具有教学资质的临床教学基地完成实习。（B 2.6.4）
- 保证毕业实习时间不少于48周，实习轮转主要安排在内科、外科、妇产科、儿科与社区。
（B 2.6.5）

- 保证在毕业实习的科室轮转安排中，内科的呼吸内科、心血管内科、消化内科分别不少于 3 周，外科的普通外科不少于 6 周，且同时包括胃肠外科和肝胆外科。（B 2.6.6）
- 在临床实践中关注患者和学生的安全。（B 2.6.7）
- 在课程计划中设置与医生职责有关的交流技能的专门指导，包括与患者及其家属或监护人、同行及其他卫生行业人员的交流等内容。（B 2.6.8）
- 安排必要的中医药课程。（B 2.6.9）
- 提倡早期接触临床。（B 2.6.10）
- 根据不同学习阶段的教学目标，合理安排临床技能的培训。（B 2.6.11）

发展标准：

医学院校应当：

- 将早期接触临床纳入课程计划，使学生更多地接触患者。（Q 2.6.1）
- 为医学生与其他专业的医疗人员及学生团队合作提供跨专业教育（IPE）的机会。（Q 2.6.2）

【注释】

- *临床医学课程包括诊断学（含检体诊断学、*

实验诊断学、影像诊断学）、外科学总论、内科学、外科学、妇产科学、儿科学、麻醉学、精神病学、神经病学、传染病学、眼科学、耳鼻咽喉科学、皮肤性病学、口腔科学、中医药学、全科医学等核心课程或内容；以及急诊医学、康复医学、老年医学等拓展课程或内容。临床医学课程也可以整合的形式呈现。核心课程与拓展课程的含义见2.4生物与基础医学课程注释。（A 2.6.1）

- *临床技能包括病史采集、体格检查、沟通技能、辅助检查、诊断与鉴别诊断、制定和执行诊疗计划、临床诊疗操作等。*（A 2.6.2）

- *合理的教学安排是指临床教学时间不少于整个课程计划时间的1/2，在临床教学中实际接触患者的时间不少于整个课程计划时间的1/3。*（A 2.6.3）

- *具有教学资质的临床教学基地是指通过教育和（或）卫生主管部门评估合格的临床教学基地。*（A 2.6.4）

- *患者和学生的安全指保证学生只承担他们能够胜任并符合相关规定的临床实践任务，并在过程中由上级医师对学生进行监督管理，*

以保护患者的安全；同时保证学生拥有安全的学习环境。（A 2.6.5）

- *早期接触临床指在生物与基础医学学习阶段，有计划地在临床环境中安排临床相关内容的学习，主要包括医患沟通、病史采集、体格检查等。*（A 2.6.6）

- *合理安排临床技能的培训指技能培训内容依据不同学习阶段设置；临床技能培训包括床旁技能训练和临床医学模拟训练。医学模拟训练是床旁教学的补充。*（A 2.6.7）

- *跨专业教育（IPE）指来自两个或多个专业的学生共同学习和有效合作，主要目标是培养学生团队合作和协同能力。*（A 2.6.8）

2.7　课程计划的结构、组成

基本标准：

医学院校必须：

- 在课程计划中简述每门课程的内容、课程安排的先后顺序以及其他课程要素，以保证人文社会科学和自然科学课程、生物与基础医学课程、公共卫生与预防医学课程和临床医学课程之间的协调。（B 2.7.1）

- 在课程设置中包括必修课程和选修课程，两

者之间的比例可根据学校的人才培养目标等实际情况确定。（B 2.7.2）

- 发挥课程教学大纲的指导作用并及时修订大纲。（B 2.7.3）

发展标准：

医学院校应当：

- 在课程计划中进行相关学科课程的不同形式的整合。（Q 2.7.1）

【注释】

- 整合包括生物与基础医学、临床医学、公共卫生与预防医学、人文社会科学等学科课程的不同形式的整合，如横向整合、纵向整合、主题模块整合等。（A 2.7.1）

2.8 课程计划管理

基本标准：

医学院校必须：

- 设置教学（指导）委员会，在教学校/院长的领导下，负责审定课程计划，以实现预期教育结果。（B 2.8.1）
- 在教学（指导）委员会中设有教师和学生代表。（B 2.8.2）
- 明确负责课程计划整体设计的部门或组织，

设置确保课程计划有效实施的基层教学组织。
（B 2.8.3）

发展标准：

医学院校应当：

- 通过教学（指导）委员会制定课程改革方案并加以实施。（Q 2.8.1）
- 在教学（指导）委员会中设有其他利益相关方的代表。（Q 2.8.2）

【注释】

- *教学（指导）委员会在学校规章制度允许范围内宏观调控课程。教学（指导）委员会有权指导教学资源的配置、推进课程计划实施、评估课程以及学生的发展情况。（A 2.8.1）*
- *其他利益相关方应该包括教学过程中的其他参与者、实习医院和其他临床机构的代表、就业单位代表、医学院校毕业生代表、社区及公众代表（如包括患者团体和组织在内的医疗服务体系的服务对象）或综合性大学的相关学院等。（A 2.8.2）*

2.9　与毕业后教育和继续医学教育的联系

基本标准：

医学院校必须：

- 确保课程计划与毕业后医学教育的有效衔接，并使毕业生具备接受继续医学教育的能力。（B 2.9.1）

发展标准：

医学院校应当：

- 根据毕业生质量调查结果和社会医疗服务需求等信息，及时修订、完善课程计划。（Q 2.9.1）

【注释】

- 有效衔接指根据医疗卫生需求，调整应达到的教育结果。有效衔接需要明确课程计划与毕业后医疗实践之间的关系；建立与卫生行政部门、用人单位、教师和学生的双向反馈机制。（A 2.9.1）

3 学业考核与评价

3.1 考核与评价方法

基本标准：

医学院校必须：

- 围绕培养目标制定并公布学生学业考核与评价的总体原则和实施方案。内容包括考核与评价的形式和频次、成绩构成、标准、允许重修次数等。（B 3.1.1）

- 确保考核与评价覆盖科学和学术、临床能力、健康与社会、职业精神与素养四个方面。（B 3.1.2）
- 根据不同的考核目的，采用合理的、多样的考核与评价方法。（B 3.1.3）
- 建立并实施考核与评价结果申诉制度。（B 3.1.4）

发展标准：

医学院校应当：

- 建立与培养目标、课程模式相适应的考核与评价的体系与方法。（Q 3.1.1）
- 积极开展考核与评价的体系与方法研究，探索新的、有效的考核与评价方法并加以应用。（Q 3.1.2）
- 确保考核与评价得到医学教育专家的指导与监督。（Q 3.1.3）

3.2 考核评价与学习之间的关系

基本标准：

医学院校必须：

- 明确采用的考核与评价原则、方法和措施，能够达到以下要求：
  - 确保学生能够实现预期的教育结果。（B 3.2.1）

- 有利于促进学生的学习。（B 3.2.2）
- 做好终结性评价的同时，加强形成性评价的应用，并及时进行反馈，以便指导学生更好地学习。（B 3.2.3）

发展标准：

医学院校应当：

- 通过调整考核与评价的频次和类型，既鼓励基础知识的掌握，又促进整合性学习。（Q 3.2.1）
- 基于考核与评价结果，及时向学生提供具有针对性和建设性的反馈意见。（Q 3.2.2）

【注释】

- 考核与评价原则、方法和措施需对应培养目标整体设计，鼓励使用客观结构化临床考试（OSCE）、微型临床评估演练（mini-CEX）、操作技能直接观察（DOPS）、计算机模拟病例考试（CCS）、置信职业行为（EPAs）评价等。（A 3.2.1）
- 终结性评价是在教学活动结束后进行，用于判断教学目标是否达到预期结果的评价手段。终结性评价侧重于学生成绩和学习结果的评定。（A 3.2.2）

- *形成性评价强调教学过程与评价过程相结合，重视和强调教与学过程中的及时反馈和改进。形成性评价既有助于教师了解教学效果并优化教学，又有助于学生及时了解自己的学习状况并调整学习策略。*（A 3.2.3）
- *整合性学习可以通过实施综合性考核来促进，同时应确保对单个学科或单门课程领域的知识进行合理覆盖。*（A 3.2.4）

3.3　考核评价结果分析与反馈

基本标准：

医学院校必须：

- 在考试完成后进行基于教育测量学的考试分析。（B 3.3.1）
- 将考核与评价的分析结果及存在的问题以适当方式反馈给学生、教师和教学管理人员。（B 3.3.2）

发展标准：

医学院校应当：

- 将考核与评价分析结果用于改进教与学。（Q 3.3.1）
- 加强考核与评价的改革与研究。（Q 3.3.2）

【注释】

- 考试分析包括试题难度和区分度、考试信度和效度、专业内容分析以及对考试整体结果的分析等。（A 3.3.1）

4　学生

4.1　招生政策及录取

基本标准：

医学院校必须：

- 根据国家的招生政策制定招生方案，并定期审核和调整。（B 4.1.1）
- 在保证招生质量的前提下，关注学生群体的多样性。（B 4.1.2）
- 在满足专业要求的前提下，不存在歧视和偏见。（B 4.1.3）
- 向社会公布招生章程及相关信息。（B 4.1.4）
- 制定并实施学生转专业的制度。（B 4.1.5）
- 具有明确的针对录取结果的申诉制度。（B 4.1.6）

发展标准：

医学院校应当：

- 阐明学生录取原则与学校宗旨、课程计划及毕业生应达到的基本要求之间的关系。（Q 4.1.1）

【注释】

- *招生章程及相关信息包括院校简介、专业设置、招生计划、收费标准、奖助学金、申诉及监督机制等方面内容，明确说明学生选拔过程并通过网络向考生公布课程计划。*（A 4.1.1）

4.2 招生规模

基本标准：

医学院校必须：

- 依据国家相关政策、社会医疗需求和学校的教育资源合理确定招生规模。（B 4.2.1）

发展标准：

医学院校应当：

- 在审核和调整招生规模时，考虑利益相关方的意见。（Q 4.2.1）
- 使招生规模体现学校办学定位与社会需求。（Q 4.2.2）

【注释】

- *社会医疗需求包括国家和区域对医学人才的需要，也包括性别、民族和其他社会需求（人群的社会文化和语言特点），如为边远地区学生及少数民族学生制定特殊招生和录取政策等。*（A 4.2.1）

- 教育资源应考虑到医学类专业学生对临床教学资源的占用。（A 4.2.2）
- 利益相关方包括教育和卫生行政部门人员、医疗卫生机构人员、教师、学生和公众代表等。（A 4.2.3）

4.3　学生咨询与支持

基本标准：

医学院校必须：

- 建立有效的学业咨询与支持体系。（B 4.3.1）
- 对学生学习、生活、勤工助学、就业等方面提供必需的支持服务。（B 4.3.2）
- 建立有效的心理咨询体系。（B 4.3.3）
- 配置学生支持服务所需的资源，关注学生事务工作队伍的建设。（B 4.3.4）
- 确保学生接受咨询与支持的隐私权不受侵犯，不泄露学生的隐私。（B 4.3.5）

发展标准：

医学院校应当：

- 根据学生学业进展情况，提供个性化学业指导和咨询。（Q 4.3.1）
- 为学生提供职业规划指导。（Q 4.3.2）

【注释】

- *学业咨询应包括课程的选择、住院医师阶段的准备等方面的内容。*（A 4.3.1）

- *支持服务包括医疗服务、就业指导、为学生（包括残障学生）提供合理的住宿，执行奖学金、贷学金、助学金、困难补助等助学制度，为学生提供经济帮助。*（A 4.3.2）

- *个性化学业指导和咨询除学习指导外，包括为每位学生或学生小组指定学术导师。*（A 4.3.3）

4.4 学生代表

基本标准：

医学院校必须：

- 制定和实施有关政策，确保学生代表能够参与课程计划的设计、管理和考核以及其他与学生有关的事宜。（B 4.4.1）

- 支持学生依法成立学生社团组织，指导和鼓励学生开展有益的社团活动，并为之提供必要的设备、场所、技术和资金支持。（B 4.4.2）

发展标准：

医学院校应当：

- 在学校的相关委员会、团体和机构中设立学生代表并发挥作用。（Q 4.4.1）

【注释】

- 学生社团组织包括学生自我管理、自我教育、自我服务的相关团体。（A 4.4.1）

5　教师

5.1　教师聘任与遴选政策

基本标准：

医学院校必须：

- 制定和实施教师资格认定制度和教师聘任制度，确保师资适应教学、科研和社会服务的需求。（B 5.1.1）

- 根据学校的目标定位、办学规模和教学模式，配备数量足够、结构合理的具有教学资质的教师队伍，尤其要确保足够数量的具有医学背景的专任教师讲授生物与基础医学相关内容。（B 5.1.2）

- 在聘任教师时应设定其职责范围，并确保其职责范围内教学、科研和社会服务之间的比例与平衡。（B 5.1.3）

- 阐明教师在教学、科研和社会服务方面的业绩标准，定期对教师的业绩进行评价。（B 5.1.4）

- 有相应的机制保证教学业绩的评价结果在职

称评定、职务晋升、岗位聘任等环节发挥作用。（B 5.1.5）

- 有相应的机制保证非医学背景教师了解医学相关知识。（B 5.1.6）

发展标准：

医学院校应当：

- 在制定教师的聘任政策时考虑学校办学宗旨、改革与发展的需求。（Q 5.1.1）
- 在制定教师的聘任政策时考虑人员经费和资源的合理有效利用，以利于教学、科研和社会服务均衡发展。（Q 5.1.2）
- 有相应的机制保证临床教师参与生物与基础医学教学。（Q 5.1.3）

【注释】

- *具有教学资质的教师*指被聘任教师必须具有良好的职业道德及与其学术等级相称的学术水平和教学能力，能够承担相应的课程和规定的教学任务，并得到相关教育部门的认可。（A 5.1.1）
- *业绩标准*可以依据教师资质、专业经验、教学奖励、科研成果、学生评价、同行评价等方面衡量。（A 5.1.2）

5.2　教师活动与教师发展政策

基本标准：

医学院校必须：

- 制定教师培训、晋升、支持和评价等政策并能有效实施，确保人才培养的中心地位。这些政策应当：
  - 保障教师的合法权利。（B 5.2.1）
  - 认可和支持教师的专业发展活动。（B 5.2.2）
  - 鼓励教师将临床经验和科研成果应用于教学。（B 5.2.3）
  - 保证教师有直接参与课程计划和教育管理决策制订的途径。（B 5.2.4）
  - 促进教师交流。（B 5.2.5）
  - 使教师具备并保持胜任教学工作的能力，鼓励教学创新。（B 5.2.6）
  - 促进教师的教学、科研和社会服务职能的平衡。（B 5.2.7）

发展标准：

医学院校应当：

- 有专门的机构或部门，制定医学教师发展规划，建立长效培训机制。（Q 5.2.1）
- 建立教师参与管理和政策制定的机制。（Q 5.2.2）

- 有相应的政策保证教师的教学、科研和社会服务职能的平衡。(Q 5.2.3)
- 保证教师对人才培养目标、课程计划有充分的了解。(Q 5.2.4)
- 有相应的机制保证承担教学任务的不同学科教师之间，特别是生物与基础医学教师和临床医学教师的相互交流与合作。(Q 5.2.5)

【注释】

- *教师活动与教师发展涉及全体教师，不仅包括新教师，也包括所有生物与基础医学教师和临床医学教师。*（A 5.2.1)
- *教师发展应重视教师教学能力的提升，为教师提供教育理念、课程设计、教学方法、教学评价等方面的培训，以及咨询、指导、技术支持与反馈。*（A 5.2.2)
- *教育管理决策还应包括招生、学生事务等。除此之外，教师也应当参与学校其他重要任务的决策。*（A 5.2.3)
- *教师对课程计划有充分的了解包括了解全部课程内容、教学方法、考核与评价方式，从而促进学科间的合作和整合，对学生进行适当的学习指导。*（A 5.2.4)

- *教师交流应包括教师在本学科领域内、学科领域间的交流，重视临床医学、生物与基础医学、公共卫生与预防医学、人文社会科学教师间的沟通交流，支持教师参加教学相关学术会议。*（A 5.2.5）

- *胜任教学工作的能力表现为能够适应学校的教育目标，遵守教学的基本原则，设计适当的教学活动和学生成绩评定方式。*（A 5.2.6）

- *教学、科研和社会服务职能的平衡指教师合理安排相关工作的时间，社会服务职能包括卫生保健系统中的临床服务、学生指导、行政管理及其他社会服务工作。*（A 5.2.7）

6 教育资源

6.1 教育经费与资源配置

基本标准：

医学院校必须：

- 有可靠的、多样化的经费筹措渠道，保证稳定的教育经费来源。（B 6.1.1）

- 有足以支持完成医学教育计划的教育经费与资源，实现培养目标。（B 6.1.2）

发展标准：

医学院校应当：

- 享有统筹使用医学教育经费与资源的自主权。（Q 6.1.1）

- 有可以支持对医学教育改革和发展探索的教育经费。（Q 6.1.2）

【注释】

- *教育经费中学校收取的学费应当按照国家有关规定管理和使用，其中教学经费及其所占学校当年财务决算的比例必须达到国家有关规定的要求。相关主管部门应保证医学教育生均拨款满足医学教育需要。学校在分配教学经费时要考虑医学教育高成本的特点。*（A 6.1.1）

- *多样化的经费筹措渠道包括政府拨款、学费收入、社会团体和公民个人投入、捐赠和基金收入、附属 / 教学医院支持、校办产业和社会服务收入等。*（A 6.1.2）

6.2 基础设施

基本标准：

医学院校必须：

- 提供足够的基础设施，确保课程计划得以有效实施。（B 6.2.1）

- 提供安全的学习环境，保证师生和患者的安全。（B 6.2.2）
- 为学生提供足够的进行临床模拟训练的场所和设备。（B 6.2.3）

发展标准：

医学院校应当：

- 定期更新、添加和拓展基础设施以改善学习、生活环境，并使其与开展的医学教育相匹配。（Q 6.2.1）
- 更新并有效利用临床模拟设备，开展临床情境的模拟教学。（Q 6.2.2）

【注释】

- *基础设施应包括各类教室及多媒体设备、小组讨论（学习）室、基础实验室（含实验设备、材料和标本）、临床技能中心及设备、临床示教室、图书馆、信息技术和网络资源，以及住宿、饮食、文体活动等设施。相关基础设施应考虑对用于教学和科研的人体标本、动物的人道关怀。（A 6.2.1）*
- 安全的学习环境指在教学实施过程中学校提供的安全学习空间，应保证师生的人身与财产安全；应提供针对有害物质、标本、微生物、植物和动物等的必要信息提示与保护措施、实验室安全条例及安全设备，并公布处理突发事件和防灾状态的制度和程序；应提供实验室安全、病原体暴露、处理危险和放射性物质等相关的必要讲解和训练。（A 6.2.2）

6.3　临床教学资源

基本标准：

医学院校必须：

- 拥有能承担全程临床教学的直属综合性三级甲等附属医院。（B 6.3.1）
- 确保足够的临床教学基地和资源，满足临床教学需要，医学类专业在校学生数与病床总数比应小于 1 ∶ 1。（B 6.3.2）
- 有足够的师资对学生的临床实践进行指导。（B 6.3.3）

发展标准：

医学院校应当：

- 持续评价、调整并更新临床教学资源，以满足教学与社会卫生服务需求。（Q 6.3.1）

【注释】

- *附属医院*是医学院校的组成部分，与学校有隶属关系。学校对附属医院主要负责人具有

任免权或附属医院党组织关系隶属于学校。（A 6.3.1）

- 临床教学基地除附属医院以外，还包括教学医院、实习医院和社区卫生实践基地。教学医院、实习医院等与学校无隶属关系。教学医院必须符合下列条件：有省级政府部门认可作为医学院校临床教学基地的资质；学校和医院双方有书面协议；有能力、有责任承担包括临床理论课、见习和实习在内的全程临床教学任务；有完善的临床教学规章制度、教学组织机构和教学团队等。（A 6.3.2）

- 临床教学资源除临床教学设施和设备之外，还包括足够的患者和病种数量。（A 6.3.3）

- 医学类专业包括临床医学、麻醉学、医学影像学、眼视光医学、精神医学、放射医学、儿科学、口腔医学、中医学、中西医临床医学、基础医学、法医学、预防医学等授予医学学士学位的专业。医学类专业在校学生包括上述专业的本科生、中/英文授课的留学生和专科生。（A 6.3.4）

- 病床总数指附属医院床位数与教学医院床位数之和，其中附属医院床位数是指参与临床教学的附属综合医院和附属专科医院的床位数之和。教学医院床位数是指承担全程临床教学并有一届临床医学专业毕业生的教学医院的床位数之和，但不包括承担部分教学的专科医院的床位数。医院的床位数为医院上一年向卫生部门呈报的年终统计报表床位数，如实际开放的床位数低于编制床位数，则按实际计算。（A 6.3.5）

- *师资既包括住院医师及以上级别的医师，也包括符合学校教学准入要求的社区医师。学校需有临床教师准入机制确保教师胜任教学。*（A 6.3.6）

- *评价临床教学资源包括对环境、设备、患者和病例病种数量、医疗卫生服务及其监督与管理等方面进行评价，衡量是否满足教学需求。还需要考虑附属医院或者教学医院承担外校医学类专业学生占用资源情况。*（A 6.3.7）

6.4 信息技术服务

基本标准：

医学院校必须：

- 拥有足够的信息技术基础设施和支持服务系统，方便学生使用。（B 6.4.1）

- 制定并实施相关政策，确保现代信息技术与资源能有效地服务于教学，保证课程计划的落实。（B 6.4.2）

发展标准：

医学院校应当：

- 保证师生能够有效利用现有的信息技术并探索新技术，以支持自主学习。（Q 6.4.1）

- 在符合医学伦理的情况下，保证学生能够最大程度地获取患者的相关病历信息及使用医疗信息系统。（Q 6.4.2）

- 在必要情况下（包括社会紧急状况），能支持将虚拟学习方法（数字、远程、分布式或在线学习）作为替代性或补充性的教学方法展开应用。（Q 6.4.3）

【注释】

- *有效利用现有的信息技术*是指通过现代信息技术手段构建校园数字化学习平台，使学生能够利用所有的教学资源，为学生利用信息技术提供支持。信息和通讯技术有助于学生自主学习和终身学习能力的培养，为学生接受未来的继续职业发展（CPD）或继续医学教育（CME）做好充分准备。（A 6.4.1）

- 分布式学习通常是在实际或虚拟地分布在不同地点的教学人员和监督人员的支持下，为在远离中心教学机构的不同地点的学生设计和开发多样的、有计划的学习课程。分布式学习是一种全体系的方法，包括所有的教与学、形成性和终结性评价、对学习的反馈、对学习者和教师的支持、管理和质量保障。分布式学习可以是整个课程计划或其中的一部分。（A 6.4.2）

6.5　教育专家

基本标准：

医学院校必须：

- 有制度和措施保证教育专家参与医学教育重要问题的决策，包括课程计划的制订，教学方法和考核与评价方式的选择、调整、改革等。（B 6.5.1）

发展标准：

医学院校应当：

- 充分发挥教育专家在教师成长中的作用。（Q 6.5.1）
- 重视培养校内教育专家的医学教育研究和评价能力。（Q 6.5.2）

【注释】

- *教育专家是指熟悉并研究医学教育问题、过程和实践且具有先进教育理念的人才，可以包括具有不同学科背景的教师、医生、管理者、研究人员等。教育专家可来自校内，也可以从其他高校或机构聘请。*（A 6.5.1）

6.6 教育交流

基本标准：

医学院校必须：

- 制定并实施与国内或国际其他教育机构合作的相关政策。（B 6.6.1）
- 提供适当资源，促进学生、教师和管理人员等进行地区间及国际间的交流。（B 6.6.2）
- 制定并实施课程学分转换的相关政策。（B 6.6.3）

发展标准：

医学院校应当：

- 考虑教师及学生的需求，尊重各方的风俗习惯和文化背景等伦理原则，有目的地组织交流活动。（Q 6.6.1）

【注释】

- *课程学分转换需在学校之间签署双方互认协*

议，确保满足本校课程计划的要求。制定公开透明的学分体系、详细描述课程要求有利于推进课程学分转换和学生交流。（A 6.6.1）

7 教育评价

7.1 教育监督与评价机制

基本标准：

医学院校必须：

- 有教育监督与评价的专职人员，并有相应机制，强调对课程计划、培养过程及结果的监督与评价。（B 7.1.1）
- 依据专业的质量标准，对教育过程各环节提出具体的要求。（B 7.1.2）
- 将相关监督与评价结果用于课程计划的改进。（B 7.1.3）
- 使学校师生与管理人员了解教育监督与评价体系。（B 7.1.4）

发展标准：

医学院校应当：

- 定期对课程计划进行全面评估，并形成周期性的报告。（Q 7.1.1）
- 对学生的学习进行跟踪评价，如学习过程、

学习能力变化、生活和学术上的支持等，并及时反馈给学生、教师、教学管理部门等利益相关方。（Q 7.1.2）

- 建有教育评价的专门机构，并能够切实发挥作用。（Q 7.1.3）
- 培训相关评价人员，使其能够选择和使用合适、有效的评价方法。（Q 7.1.4）

【注释】

- *教育评价*指根据相应的标准，运用科学手段，通过系统地收集信息资料和分析整理，对课程计划、培养过程和结果进行质量判断，为提高教育质量和教育决策提供依据的过程。信息资料可包括政策、规章制度、会议纪要、与其他教育机构的联合协议等；还可包括本科医学教育质量报告以及学生、教师、督导、外部专家、用人单位、主管部门等利益相关方关于教育教学的评价数据和结果。（A 7.1.1）
- *教育监督*指针对课程主要环节的观察和督导，包括日常资料收集等，目的在于保证教育活动的正常运行，并及时发现需要干预的环节。这种信息收集往往是与招生、学生考核与评价、毕业等相关联的行政管理过程的一

部分。（A 7.1.2）

- *周期性的报告包括实施教学的环境、课程计划的具体内容和实施、培养结果和社会责任的体现等。实施教学的环境包括医学院校的组织制度环境、资源环境、学习环境和文化氛围。培养结果可通过校内外组织的考试 [如各阶段综合考试、医学院校临床医学专业（本科）水平测试、国家临床执业医师资格考试、住院医师规范化培训结业考试等]、职业选择、就业去向、毕业后表现等来反映，可作为本科医学教育改进的参考。（A 7.1.3）*

7.2　教师和学生反馈

基本标准：

医学院校必须：

- 采用多种评价方式，系统地搜集信息，分析教师和学生的反馈并做出回复。（B 7.2.1）

发展标准：

医学院校应当：

- 将反馈结果用于课程计划的改进并取得成效。（Q 7.2.1）

【注释】

- 反馈不仅包括教育过程、教育结果方面的信

息，还应包括学校的政策措施、教师和学生的各种违纪行为的处理等。（A 7.2.1）

7.3 学生表现

基本标准：

医学院校必须：

- 将学生在校期间和毕业后的表现与学校办学宗旨、预期教育结果、课程计划和提供的教育资源联系起来。（B 7.3.1）

发展标准：

医学院校应当：

- 将学生发展和毕业生质量的分析结果作为制定招生政策、课程计划修订、学生咨询服务的依据。（Q 7.3.1）

【注释】

- 学生在校期间和毕业后的表现可通过采集和使用各种教育结果数据，表明教育目标完成的程度进行体现。（A 7.3.1）
- 学生发展包括在校生的身心发展和学业发展。学业发展的测量和分析包括学习期限、考试分数、考试通过率、学业完成率和辍学率等。学校可通过问卷调查、座谈会、学业成就数据分析等方式对学生发展做教育增值评价。（A 7.3.2）

- *毕业生质量的分析应围绕毕业生基本要求的内容进行，包括毕业生的职业选择、临床实践的表现和晋升等信息的收集、整理和分析。*（A 7.3.3）

7.4　利益相关方的参与

基本标准：

医学院校必须：

- 有教师、学生和行政管理部门人员等校内利益相关方参与教育监督与评价。（B 7.4.1）

发展标准：

医学院校应当：

- 鼓励校外利益相关方参与对课程计划的监督与评价，了解评估的结果。（Q 7.4.1）
- 征询校外利益相关方对毕业生质量、课程计划的反馈意见。（Q 7.4.2）

【注释】

- *校外利益相关方包括其他学术和管理人员代表、社区和公众代表（如医疗服务的对象）、教育和卫生行政部门以及医疗卫生机构和毕业后教育工作者等。*（A 7.4.1）

8 科学研究

8.1 教学与科学研究

基本标准：

医学院校必须：

- 制定并实施相关政策，促进科研与教学协调发展。（B 8.1.1）
- 加强对医学教育及管理的研究，为教学改革与发展提供理论依据。（B 8.1.2）

发展标准：

医学院校应当：

- 将科研活动、科研成果引入教学过程，以培养学生的科学方法、科学思维及科学精神，保证科学研究和教学之间的良性互动。（Q 8.1.1）
- 建立专门的医学教育研究机构，在推进医学教育改革、提高教师的教育科学研究能力方面切实发挥作用。（Q 8.1.2）

【注释】

- 医学教育研究是指根据相关理论针对医学教育活动开展的教育科学研究，主要对医学教育理论、实践和社会层面的问题进行研究，目的是深入揭示医学教育规律，为医学教育

改革提供理论与研究支撑。（A 8.1.1）

8.2 教师科研

基本标准：

医学院校必须：

- 为教师提供基本的科学研究条件，鼓励教师开展科学研究，促进科研与教学相结合。（B 8.2.1）
- 要求教师具备相应的科学研究能力。（B 8.2.2）

发展标准：

医学院校应当：

- 有相应机制保证教师参与医学教育研究，提升教学能力。（Q 8.2.1）

8.3 学生科研

基本标准：

医学院校必须：

- 将科学研究活动作为培养学生科学素养和创新思维的重要途径，采取积极、有效的措施为学生创造参与科学研究的机会与条件。（B 8.3.1）
- 在课程计划中安排综合性、设计性实验，开设学术讲座、组织科研小组等，开展有利于培养学生科研能力的活动。（B 8.3.2）

- 使学生了解医学科学研究的基本方法和伦理原则。（B 8.3.3）

发展标准：

医学院校应当：

- 为学生提供科学研究经费，以满足学生参与科学研究的需要。（Q 8.3.1）

9　管理与行政

9.1　管理体制与机制

基本标准：

医学院校必须：

- 明确阐述学校、医学院及附属医院之间的管理体制与结构，界定学校、医学院及附属医院的管理职能，建立学校、医学院及附属医院之间的有效管理机制，保证医学教育的完整性，确保教学的有效运行和可持续发展。（B 9.1.1）
- 设立相应委员会，审议课程计划、教学改革及科学研究等重要事项。委员会应该包括院校领导、师生代表和管理人员等校内利益相关方代表。（B 9.1.2）

发展标准：

医学院校应当：

- 在相应委员会中包含上级行政主管部门、医疗卫生机构及社会公众等校外利益相关方代表。（Q 9.1.1）
- 保证医学教育管理工作和决策过程的透明性。（Q 9.1.2）

【注释】

- *管理*主要涉及政策制定、决策过程及政策执行的监管。学校政策和教育教学政策通常涵盖医学办学宗旨、课程计划、招生政策、员工招聘与选拔等方面的规定以及与医疗卫生部门及其他校外机构的联系与合作方面的决策。（A 9.1.1）
- *委员会*组成人员应有广泛的代表性。委员会的活动应明确组织者或召集人，相关人员参与活动的时间、内容应有记录。（A 9.1.2）
- *透明性*可通过简讯、网络信息和会议报道等方式得以实现。（A 9.1.3）

9.2 医学教育主管领导

基本标准：

医学院校必须：

- 明确阐述医学教育主管领导对医学教育的管理职责和在人财物等方面的权限，并确保有效执行。（B 9.2.1）
- 重视医学教育主管领导的专业背景。（B 9.2.2）
- 保证医学教育管理部门领导任职时间相对稳定。（B 9.2.3）

发展标准：

医学院校应当：

- 定期评估医学教育主管领导在教学管理过程中的业绩。（Q 9.2.1）

【注释】

- *医学教育主管领导包括医学教育主要负责领导及管理部门中负责教学、科研和服务等方面学术事宜决策的人员。*（A 9.2.1）

9.3 行政人员及管理

基本标准：

医学院校必须：

- 配齐医学教育管理队伍人员，建立结构合理、理念先进的行政管理队伍，确保医学教育的

顺利实施。（B 9.3.1）

- 建立科学的管理制度及操作程序，确保资源合理配置。（B 9.3.2）
- 有相应措施保证医学教育管理人员理解医学教育并了解医学教育全过程。（B 9.3.3）

发展标准：

医学院校应当：

- 定期评价并改进医学教育管理工作。（Q 9.3.1）

9.4 与医疗卫生机构、行政管理部门的相互关系

基本标准：

医学院校必须：

- 与行政管理部门加强联系和交流，争取各方面对人才培养的支持。（B 9.4.1）
- 与相关医疗卫生机构签署协议，保证教学的顺利实施。（B 9.4.2）

发展标准：

医学院校应当：

- 与医疗卫生机构和行政管理部门开展更广泛的合作与交流，保证合作与交流的可持续发展。（Q 9.4.1）

【注释】

- *相关医疗卫生机构除包含公立或私立医疗服*

务机构、医学研究机构之外，还包含健康促进组织、疾病防控机构等。（A 9.4.1）

- 广泛的合作与交流指达成正式协议，明确合作的内容与形式并开展合作项目等。（A 9.4.2）

10　改革与发展

基本标准：

医学院校必须：

- 对医学教育教学改革进行系统设计，展开循证研究，并对改革的效果进行科学评价。（B 10.0.1）
- 建立相应机制，定期回顾和评估自身发展，明确自身存在的问题并持续改进。（B 10.0.2）

发展标准：

医学院校应当：

- 基于前瞻性研究、医学教育文献研究、各类评估评价结果等不断反思，持续改进。（Q 10.0.1）
- 通过改革形成相应的政策和措施，并与既往经验、现状和未来发展相适应。（Q 10.0.2）
- 基于卫生健康需求变化、社会与科技发展趋势，调整教育策略。（Q 10.0.3）

Standards for Basic Medical Education in China

The 2022 Revision

Working Committee for the Accreditation of Medical Education, Ministry of Education, P. R. China

Contents

Preface

Medical education programs in China carry out the mission of training competent health professionals, thusly closely related to the health outcomes of all citizens. Since the Ministry of Education (MOE) and the former Ministry of Health issued *Standards for Basic Medical Education (for Trial Implementation)* in 2008, the accreditation system of basic medical education in China has been gradually developed. The Working Committee for the Accreditation of Medical Education (WCAME) of the MOE has been established, the official *Guidelines for Accreditation of Medical Education (for Trial Implementation)* has been released, and the accreditation activities have been steadily conducted. In 2016, WCAME officially released *Standards for Basic Medical Education in China (The 2016 Revision)*, which was used as the basis for a new round of accreditation.

In June 2020, WCAME was officially recognized by the World Federation for Medical Education (WFME), marking that China's medical education standards and accreditation system have achieved international substantive equivalence, and the quality of medical education accreditation has been internationally recognized. By the end of 2021, WCAME had completed the first round of accreditation of basic medical education in China.

In order to ensure that the medical education standards keep pace with the times and better promote the new round of accreditation, WCAME summarized the beneficial experience of accreditation for basic medical education in China, timely introduced the latest concepts of medical education, started the revision of the 2016 Standards in 2021, and formed *Standards for Basic Medical Education in China (The 2022 Revision)*.

The 2022 revision is still composed of two parts: graduate outcomes of basic medical education, and standards for basic medical education in China. In standards for basic medical education in China, it still incorporates at two levels of attainment, the basic standards (B) and quality development standards (Q). The basic standard in principle must be met by every medical school providing basic medical education, which is expressed with a "must" statement. The quality development standard is in accordance with international consensus on the best practices in basic medical education hereby representing the trend of development, which is expressed with a "should" statement. Fulfillment of quality development standards will vary with the phases of development, available resources, educational policy and other conditions of the medical schools. Compared with the 2016 revision, the set of standards in the 2022 revision is still grouped into 10 main areas and 40 sub-areas; the original 113 basic standards and 80 quality development standards were adjusted to 117 basic standards and 76 quality development standards. At the same time, to enhance the readability, we adopt a digital index for the annotations (A) with a total of 86 items.

The 2022 revision, applicable to basic medical education in China, serves as the basis for its accreditation. As the first stage of the continuum of medical education, basic medical education is to develop a medical graduate with foundational clinical ability, life-long learning capability and desired quality of professionalism through complete medical training processes. It lays an essential foundation for postgraduate medical education and practice in various health care institutions for the medical students. The professional capability of basic medical graduates in clinical practices needs to be gradually formed and improved in the postgraduate medical education, the continuing professional development and the continuing medical practices.

The 2022 revision reflects the international trend, taking consideration of the domestic needs and societal expectations of medical education systems in China, which is the basis for formulating educational programs and standardizing educational management. Each medical school is required to determine its educational objectives, formulate its expected educational outcomes and curriculum, and establish its program evaluation system and quality assurance mechanism based on its own characteristics and standards in the 2022 revision.

The revision also acknowledges the differences in geographic locations and among institutions, and respects the autonomy of each medical school. With the prerequisite of adhering to the basic principles of medical education, the revision does not set many specific and compulsory requirements to educational program apart from essential ones, so that there is sufficient space for the development and operations of each institution. It should be highlighted that these standards implement the education policy of the country, strengthen morality education of talents, and are committed to guiding the practice of medical education in China, so as to improve the quality of medical talent training.

Graduate outcomes of basic medical education

The graduates of basic medical education in China should develop the correct views of the world, life and values. They should possess core values of patriotism and collectivism, and be loyal to the people. Besides abiding by the law, they should be willing to make a lifetime dedication to the development of the health care service of the country and the physical and mental well-being of mankind.

The graduate outcomes of basic medical education in China are presented in four domains: Science and Scholarship, Clinical Practice, Health and Society, and Professionalism. More specific requirements of the expected outcomes should be formulated by each institution on the basis of actual situation.

Medical education is a continuum covering basic education, postgraduate education and continuing professional development. At the end of basic medical education, the graduates will possess corresponding foundations for medical practice. However, the graduates do not have rich clinical experiences upon graduation, which requires them to keep upgrading their professional competence in time with the advancing pace in medicine. The education and training graduates obtained and scientific methods they acquired in school will provide support for their lifelong learning and development.

1. Science and Scholarship: the medical graduate as a scientist and a scholar

At the end of basic medical education, graduates are able to:

1.1   Possess the fundamental knowledge of the disciplines such as natural sciences, humanities and social sciences and medicine, and apply scientific methods, which will be applicable in future study and medical practices.

1.2   Apply medical and other scientific knowledge to deal with medical or health related problems in individuals, populations and health systems.

1.3   Understand and describe the prevention and etiology, pathology, course, clinical manifestations, diagnosis, treatment, outcome, prognosis and rehabilitation of diseases at all stages of life.

1.4　Master the basic features of traditional Chinese medicine and its basic principle of diagnosis and treatment.

1.5　Access, critically appraise, interpret and apply evidence from the medical and scientific literature.

1.6　Apply knowledge of common scientific methods to formulate relevant research questions.

2．Clinical Practice：the medical graduate as a practitioner

At the end of basic medical education, graduates are able to:

2.1　Conduct effective communications with patients, their family members or guardians, colleagues and health professionals of other disciplines.

2.2　Take a medical history in a proper, comprehensive and systematic way.

2.3　Perform a full and accurate physical examination, including a mental state examination, and write medical records as required.

2.4   Integrate and interpret findings from the medical history and examination, to arrive at an initial assessment including a relevant differential diagnosis. Discriminate between possible differential diagnoses and propose rational management principles.

2.5   Select and justify common investigations, with regard to the pathological basis of disease, utility, safety and cost effectiveness, and interpret the results.

2.6   Select and perform common procedures safely.

2.7   Make clinical judgements and decisions based on available evidence. Identify and justify relevant treatment options under the guidance of supervising physicians.

2.8   Understand patients' questions, views, concerns and preferences, and ensure patients and their families or guardians' full understanding of their situations and options. Communicate on the risks and benefits of treatment options, and involve patients and their families or guardians in the decision-making and planning of their treatments (shared decision-making).

2.9   Provide information to patients, and their families or guardians where relevant, to enable them to make fully informed choices among various diagnostic, therapeutic and treatment options.

2.10　Apply prevention, early detection, health maintenance and chronic disease management where relevant to clinical practices.

2.11　Propose safe, effective, and economical treatment options based on objective evidence.

2.12　Recognise and evaluate changes in the patient's condition and its severity, and to provide possible emergency treatment for patients requiring urgent care.

2.13　Master the principles of end-of-life care for patients and communicate with patients and their families or guardians. Use symptomatic, psychological support and other palliative treatment methods to achieve humanitarian purposes, so as to improve the quality of death.

2.14　Retrieve, interpret and record information effectively in clinical information systems.

3. Health and Society: the medical graduate as a health advocate

At the end of basic medical education, graduates are able to:

3.1　Have responsibility to protect and advance the

health and well-being of individuals and populations.

3.2   Understand factors that contribute to health, diagnosis and effective treatment of populations, including issues relating to health equalities, diversity of cultural and community values, and socio-economic and physical environment.

3.3   Communicate effectively with wider roles in various situation, such as doctors, health advocates, researchers, etc.

3.4   Explain and evaluate common population health screening and prevention approaches, including the use of technology for surveillance and monitoring of the health status of populations, and provide instructions on patients' follow-up visits, medications and rehabilitative therapies, etc.

3.5   Understand the quality assurance system and safety management system of health care in hospitals, and be aware of their own competence, responsibility and limits in medical practice. Attach importance to patients' safety, and recognize relevant risk factors in time.

3.6   Understand the structures and functions of the national health care system in China, and the roles and relationships between health agencies and services, and understand the principles of rational allocation of resources, to meet the needs of individuals, populations and national health systems.

3.7　Understand the global health issues and the affecting factors of health and diseases.

4．Professionalism: the medical graduate as a professional

At the end of basic medical education, graduates are able to:

4.1　Provide humanistic and quality health care services to all patients in accordance with the *Ethic Principles of Chinese Physicians*.

4.2　Demonstrate professional values in health practice, including empathy, respect for all patients and commitment to high quality clinical service standards, and form personal qualities of honest, integrity, teamwork and leadership.

4.3　Master and apply the main principles of medical ethics in clinical practices. Communicate effectively with patients and their family members or guardians, colleagues and other health care professionals regarding ethical issues in medicine.

4.4   Be aware of the factors affecting physicians' health and wellbeing, such as fatigue, stress management and infection control, to mitigate health risks of professional practice, and identify the potential risks posed to patients by their own health.

4.5   Abide by the laws and regulations regarding clinical practice as well as professional ethics.

4.6   Recognize the limits of their own expertise, and show respect for other health care professionals, to learn and work effectively as a team.

4.7   Demonstrate awareness of self-directed learning and lifelong learning. Recognize the importance of continuous self-improvement and demonstrate a commitment to excellence.

Standards for Basic Medical Education in China

1. Mission and Outcomes

1.1 Mission

Basic standards:

The medical school **must**

- state its mission and make it known to its stakeholders including the leadership, staff and students of the school and health sectors and etc. (B 1.1.1)

- elaborate the overall objectives and the implementation of educational strategy in its mission, to make sure its medical graduates meet the graduate outcomes of basic medical education. (B 1.1.2)

- on the premise of abiding by relevant laws, consider that the mission encompasses the health needs of the community, the needs of the health care system and other aspects of social accountability. (B 1.1.3)

Quality development standards:

The medical school **should**

- ensure that the mission encompasses:
    - orientation of medical research. (Q 1.1.1)
    - requirements for the concepts of one health and aspects of global health. (Q 1.1.2)

Annotations:

- *Mission* illustrates the overarching framework of medical education of a medical school, including its positioning, educational philosophy and expected outcomes. It should match the resources and management of the school, while taking into consideration the local and national, regional and global expectations of medicine and the needs of development. It should also reflect the history, culture, and the development vision of the school. The positioning of the school should reflect its purpose, type and level of the education it provides, the community it serves and its development goals. The educational philosophy should reflect the concepts and ideas it upholds in the training of medical students. (A 1.1.1)

- *The Medical school* is the educational institution offering basic medical education programs. The medical school can be an independent institution or part of or affiliated to a university. Medical schools would include university affiliated hospitals and other affiliated clinical facilities. Medical school not only provides basic medical education, medical research and medical services but also provides educational programs for other stages of medical education and for other health professions. (A 1.1.2)

- *Encompassing the health needs of the community* refers to interaction with the local community, especially the health and health related sectors, and adjustment of the curriculum to demonstrate attention to and knowledge about health problems of the community. (A 1.1.3)

- *Social accountability* refers to the willingness and ability to respond to the needs of society, of patients and the health and health related sectors and to contribute to the national and global development of medicine by fostering competencies in health care, medical education and medical research. This would be based on the autonomy of the school. In matters outside its control especially health related issues, the medical school would still demonstrate social accountability by explaining relationships and drawing attention to consequences. (A 1.1.4)

- *Medical research* would include basic biomedical sciences, clinical sciences and skills, public health and preventive medicine sciences and other medical related scientific research. (A 1.1.5)

- *Aspects of global health* refers to the awareness of major global health priorities and concerns in different regions, including awareness of major international health problems, and of health consequences of inequality and injustice due to racial differences, regional and wealth disparity, and of cross-disciplinary, cross-sector and cross-border health management to address above challenges. (A 1.1.6)

1.2　Participation in formulation of mission

Basic standard:

The medical school **must**

- ensure that its principal stakeholders on campus participate in formulating the mission. (B 1.2.1)

Quality development standard:

The medical school **should**

- have a mechanism for its stakeholders off campus to participate in the formulation of the mission and effectively implement it. (Q 1.2.1)

Annotations:

- *Principal stakeholders on campus* would include teachers, students, leadership and administrative staff of a university/school. (A 1.2.1)

- *Stakeholders off campus* would include representatives of education and health care authorities, employers, the community and public (e.g., users of the health care delivery system, including patient organizations), academic and administrative staff, professional organizations, medical scientific bodies and postgraduate educators. (A 1.2.2)

1.3   Institutional autonomy and academic freedom

Basic standards:

The medical school **must**

- have the autonomy to formulate and implement policies in compliance with relevant laws and regulations, especially regarding
  - design of the curriculum. (B 1.3.1)
  - allocation and use of the resources necessary for implementation of the curriculum. (B 1.3.2)
- obtain the academic support of medical education from the disciplines such as natural sciences, humanities and social sciences. (B 1.3.3)
- ensure academic freedom for its academic staff/ faculty and students. (B 1.3.4)

Quality development standard:

The medical school **should**

- enhance the integration of humanities, social and natural sciences with the medical sciences. (Q 1.3.1)

Annotations:

- *Institutional autonomy* would include appropriate independence from government and other counterparts (regional and local authorities, private co-operations, the professions, unions and other interest groups) to be able to make decisions in key areas such as student admission, design of curriculum, assessments, staff recruitment/selection and employment conditions, research and resource allocation. Institutional autonomy should be respected on the premise of complying with national laws and regulations and the developmental principles of medical education. (A 1.3.1)
- *Academic freedom* should be respected on the premise of complying national laws and regulations. (A 1.3.2)

1.4   Educational outcomes

Basic standards:

The medical school **must**

- define the intended educational outcomes that students should exhibit upon graduation in relation to science and scholarship, clinical practice, health and society, and professionalism, and clarify the educational outcomes that are consistent with the school's mission. (B 1.4.1)

- ensure appropriate student conducts with respect to fellow students, faculty members, other health care professionals, patients and their families or guardians. (B 1.4.2)

Quality development standards:

The medical school **should**

- specify and co-ordinate the linkage of outcomes to be acquired by graduation with acquired outcomes in postgraduate training. (Q 1.4.1)
- specify requirements for and expected outcomes of student engagement in medical research. (Q 1.4.2)
- specify requirements for students' understanding of one health and global health. (Q 1.4.3)

Annotation:

- *Educational outcomes* can be measured and evaluated by corresponding means, such as academic assessment, student comprehensive evaluation, student development and graduate survey, employment and career development analysis, etc. Academic assessment includes curricular assessment, graduation assessment, the Level Test of Basic Medical Education (undergraduate) in Medical Schools, the National Medical Licensing Examination (NMLE), etc. (A 1.4.1)

2．Curriculum

2.1　Curriculum design and implementation

Basic standards:

The medical school **must**

- make its curriculum suitable for the mission, objectives and educational outcomes of the school, which based upon the medical and health needs of the community and society, the advances in medical sciences and the transforming trends of healthcare services. (B 2.1.1)

- ensure that the curriculum upholds the principles of strengthening foundational learning and skills training, emphasizing professionalism and personal quality development. (B 2.1.2)

- define the curriculum models. (B 2.1.3)
- define the suitable instructional and learning methods employed, which is based upon different curricular objectives, contents and teaching objects. (B 2.1.4)
- ensure that the curriculum and instructional/learning methods could stimulate, prepare and support students to take responsibility for their self-directed learning. (B 2.1.5)
- ensure that the curriculum is delivered in accordance with principles of equality. (B 2.1.6)

Quality development standards:

The medical school **should**

- have a scientific and systematic design and implementation of the fostering of students' self-directed learning and lifelong learning ability. (Q 2.1.1)
- reflect the new trend of scientific development in the curriculum. (Q 2.1.2)

Annotations:

- *Curriculum* in this document refers to the educational program and it includes a statement of the training objectives, intended educational outcomes, curriculum models, experiences and processes of the program (consisting of a description of the course structure and composition, credit hours and time allocation), assessment principles, etc. The curriculum shall have a matched curriculum syllabus. The syllabus covers the teaching objectives, teaching contents, instructional and learning methods, learning resources, assessment requirements and other contents of the course. Each part of the syllabus should coordinate with each other and adapt to the training objectives. (A 2.1.1)

- *Curriculum models* would include models based on disciplines, or various integration. (A 2.1.2)

- *Instructional and learning methods* encompass lectures, small-group teaching, problem-based and case-based learning, peer assisted learning, laboratory teaching, clinical demonstrations, bedside teaching, clinical skills laboratory training, situational teaching, simulation/virtual teaching, online and offline hybrid teaching, etc. (A 2.1.3)

- *Self-directed learning* refers to a kind of learning behavior that learners are driving themselves, judging their own learning needs, formulating suitable learning goals, identifying and integrating relevant learning content and resources, selecting appropriate learning methods and strategies, monitoring their own learning process, evaluating their own learning effects, and constantly adjusting themselves. (A 2.1.4)

- *Principles of equality* refers to that schools abide by the principles of fairness and diversity in the implementation of teaching. The gender, ethnicity, religion and socio-economic status of students shall be fully considered when formulating rules and regulations on teaching management and student evaluation. (A 2.1.5)

- The *curriculum and instructional and learning methods* would be based on contemporary learning principles. (A 2.1.6)

2.2　Scientific method

Basic standards:

The medical school **must**

- throughout the curriculum teach
  - the principles of scientific methods, including the ability to analyze and solve problems and critical thinking. (B 2.2.1)
  - medical research methods. (B 2.2.2)
  - evidence-based medicine. (B 2.2.3)

Quality development standards:

The medical school **should**

- encourage and support students to participate in research projects and include scientific research training throughout the curriculum. (Q 2.2.1)
- include elements of original or advanced research in the curriculum. (Q 2.2.2)
- integrate scientific principles, medical research method and innovation awareness throughout the curriculum. (Q 2.2.3)

Annotation:

- *Scientific method* refers to the fostering of

scientific methods and scientific consciousness in the curriculum. (A 2.2.1)

2.3   Humanities and social sciences and natural sciences

Basic standards:

The medical school **must**

- in the curriculum identify and incorporate the contributions of:
  - humanities and social sciences, especially ideological morality, medical ethics, health laws and regulations, etc. (B 2.3.1)
  - natural sciences. (B 2.3.2)

Quality development standards:

The medical school **should**

- integrate humanities and social sciences into medical education, with emphasis on professionalism, in the curriculum adjust and modify the contributions of the humanities and social sciences to:
  - scientific, technological and clinical developments. (Q 2.3.1)
  - current and anticipated needs of the society

and the health care system. (Q 2.3.2)

- changing demographic and cultural contexts. (Q 2.3.3)

Annotations:

- *Humanities and social sciences* include history of medicine, medical ethics, medical jurisprudence, medical psychology, medical sociology, health services administration, etc. Its content and depth depend on program objectives. The medical school is encouraged to integrate humanities and social sciences effectively into the course contents of medical disciplines or other professional trainings. (A 2.3.1)

- *Natural sciences* include mathematics, physics and chemistry, etc. (A 2.3.2)

2.4　Basic biomedical sciences

Basic standard:

The medical school **must**

- in the curriculum identify and incorporate the contributions of the basic biomedical sciences to create understanding of scientific knowledge, concepts and methods fundamental to acquiring and their applying in clinical practice. (B 2.4.1)

Quality development standard:

The medical school **should**

- in the curriculum adjust and modify the contributions of the basic biomedical sciences to the scientific, technological and clinical developments as well as current and anticipated needs of the society and the health care system. (Q 2.4.1)

Annotation:

- *Basic biomedical sciences* would include core courses or contents like human anatomy (include systematic anatomy and regional anatomy), histology and embryology, cell biology, medical genetics, biochemistry and molecular biology, physiology, pathogenic biology, medical immunology, pathology, pharmacology, pathophysiology and developing courses or contents which related with medical discipline development like neurobiology. All the above courses or contents can also be presented in the form of integration. Core courses or contents are always compulsory and developing courses or contents can be compulsory or elective based on program objectives and the schools' resources. (A 2.4.1)

2.5　Public health and preventive medicine sciences

Basic standard:

The medical school **must**

- in the curriculum identify and incorporate the contributions of public health and preventive medicine sciences to develop students' awareness of population health and disease prevention strategies, allowing them to function well in health education, promotion and management efforts, and to apply these knowledge and skills in clinical practice. (B 2.5.1)

Quality development standards:

The medical school **should**

- integrate public health and preventive medicine into the whole process of medical education. (Q 2.5.1)
- ensure that the curriculum expands the students'

vision in global health, so the learners understand the global health issues and think in global health perspectives. (Q 2.5.2)

Annotation:

- *Public health and preventive medicine sciences* include medical statistics, epidemiology, maternal and child health care, child and adolescent health, social medicine, environmental hygiene, nutrition and food hygiene, occupational health and occupational medicine, global health, health promotion and health education, etc. (A 2.5.1)

2.6   Clinical sciences and skills

Basic standards:

The medical school **must**

- in the curriculum identify and incorporate the contributions of the clinical sciences to ensure that students acquire sufficient clinical science knowledge and clinical skill, and professionalism to assume appropriate responsibilities after graduation. (B 2.6.1)

- ensure that students spend a reasonable part of the program in planned contact with patients in relevant clinical settings. (B 2.6.2)

- ensure the effective integration of medical knowledge and clinical clerkship. (B 2.6.3)

- ensure that each student completes his or her internship at affiliated hospital of the medical school and the clinical site that has written agreement with the medical school and possesses appropriate teaching qualifications. (B 2.6.4)

- satisfy the time requirement of clinical internship prior to graduation, which is no less than 48 weeks, and the rotation is mainly arranged in internal medicine, surgery, gynecology and obstetrics, pediatrics and community. (B 2.6.5)

- ensure that the time students spend on the rotation shall not be less than 3 weeks in respiratory medicine, cardiovascular medicine and digestive medicine of internal medicine respectively, and shall not be less than 6 weeks in general surgery including gastrointestinal surgery and hepatobiliary surgery of surgery. (B 2.6.6)

- organize clinical trainings with appropriate attention to patient and student safety. (B 2.6.7)

- in the curriculum identify and incorporate the contributions of communication skills related with the doctors' responsibilities to ensure that students communicate professionally with patients, their families or guardians, peers and other medical team members. (B 2.6.8)
- include necessary traditional Chinese medicine courses in the curriculum. (B 2.6.9)
- encourage early clinical exposure. (B 2.6.10)
- structure different elements of clinical skills training reasonably according to the teaching objectives of different phases in the program. (B 2.6.11)

Quality development standards:

The medical school **should**

- include early clinical exposure into the curriculum, so as to allow students to contact patients more. (Q 2.6.1)
- provide students opportunities for interprofessional education (IPE) to work with medical professionals and student teams from other specialties. (Q 2.6.2)

Annotations:

- *The clinical sciences* would include core courses or contents like diagnostics (including physical diagnostics, laboratory diagnostics, imaging diagnostics), internal medicine, surgery, gynecology, obstetrics, pediatrics, anesthesiology, psychiatry, neurological diseases, infectious diseases, ophthalmology, otolaryngology, dermatovenerology, stomatology, traditional Chinese medicine and pharmacy and general practice/family medicine; and developing courses or contents like emergency medicine, rehabilitation, geriatrics. The courses for clinical medicine can also be presented in the form of integration. Refer to 2.4 (basic biomedical sciences) for the meanings of core courses and developing courses. (A 2.6.1)

- *Clinical skills* include history taking, physical examination, communication skills, auxiliary examination, diagnosis and differentiated diagnosis, clinical procedural performance, prescription and treatment practices, etc. (A 2.6.2)

- *A reasonable part* would mean the fact that the clinical teaching time is no less than half of the program and that the contact with patients in the clinical settings accounts for no less than one third of the program. (A 2.6.3)

- *Clinical teaching sites with teaching qualification* indicate qualified teaching hospitals that have been accredited by education and/or health authorities. (A 2.6.4)

- *Patient and student safety* would require close supervision of clinical activities conducted by students under superior physician to ensure the patients' safety and provide safe learning environment for students. (A 2.6.5)

- *Early clinical exposure* would partly take place in primary care settings and would primarily include history taking, physical examination and communication with patients, families and healthcare professionals. (A 2.6.6)

- *Structure different elements of clinical skills training reasonably* means that the content of skill training is set according to different learning phases; Clinical skill training includes bedside skill training and simulated clinical training. Simulated clinical training is a supplement to bedside teaching. (A 2.6.7)

- *Interprofessional education (IPE)* refers to the joint learning and effective cooperation of students from two or more majors, which mainly aims at developing students' ability of teamwork and collaboration. (A 2.6.8)

2.7　Curriculum structure, composition and duration

Basic standards:

The medical school **must**

- sketch the content, extent and sequencing of courses and other curricular elements to ensure appropriate coordination among humanities and social, natural, basic biomedical, public health and preventive medicine and clinical subjects. (B 2.7.1)

- include elective courses in curriculum and define the balance between the core and elective courses according to school's talent training objectives. (B 2.7.2)

- give play to the guiding role of the curriculum syllabus and revise the syllabus in a timely manner. (B 2.7.3)

Quality development standard:

The medical school **should**

- conduct integration of related discipline courses in the curriculum in different forms. (Q 2.7.1)

Annotation:

- *Integration* could be different forms of integration of basic biomedical sciences, clinical sciences, public health and preventive medicine sciences, humanities and social sciences and other disciplines. Examples of integration could be horizontal integration, vertical integration, and thematic blocks integration. (A 2.7.1)

2.8   Curriculum management

Basic standards:

The medical school **must**

- have a curriculum committee, which is under the governance of the academic leadership (the Dean) responsible for reviewing the curriculum to secure its intended educational outcomes. (B 2.8.1)

- in its curriculum committee ensure proper representation of staff and students. (B 2.8.2)
- specify the department or organization responsible for the overall design of the curriculum and set up grassroots teaching organizations to ensure the effective implementation of the curriculum. (B 2.8.3)

Quality development standards:

The medical school **should**

- through its curriculum committee plan and implement innovations in the curriculum. (Q 2.8.1)
- in its curriculum committee include representatives of other stakeholders. (Q 2.8.2)

Annotations:

- The authority of the *curriculum committee* would include the control of the curriculum within existing rules and regulations. The curriculum committee would allocate the granted resources for planning and implementing of the curriculum and evaluation of courses, as well as the evaluation of student development. (A 2.8.1)

- *Other stakeholders* would include other participants in the educational process, representing the teaching hospitals, clinical facilities, employer, alumni, other health professions or faculties in the University. Other stakeholders might also include groups representing the community and public (e.g., users of the healthcare delivery system, including patient organizations). (A 2.8.2)

2.9   Linkage with postgraduate medical education and continuing medical education

Basic standard:

The medical school **must**

- ensure operational linkage between the educational program and the subsequent stages of training or practice after graduation, making it possible for the graduates to receive continuing medical education. (B 2.9.1)

Quality development standard:

The medical school **should**

- ensure that the curriculum committee seeks

input from institutions in which graduates will be expected to work, and modify the program accordingly, and considers program modification in response to feedback from the community and society. (Q 2.9.1)

Annotation:

- *The operational linkage* implies identifying healthcare needs and defining required educational outcomes. This requires clear definition and description of the elements within the educational programs and their inter-relationships with training and practice after graduating, paying attention to the local, national, regional and global context. It would include mutual feedback to and from the health sector and participation of teachers and students in activities of the health team. Operational linkage also implies constructive dialogue with potential employers of the graduates as the basis for career guidance. (A 2.9.1)

3. Assessment and Evaluation of Students

3.1 Assessment and evaluation methods

Basic standards:

The medical school **must**

- define, state and publish the principles, methods and practices used for assessment and evaluation of its students, including the type and frequency of assessment and evaluation, composition of marks, criteria, number of allowed retakes, etc. (B 3.1.1)

- ensure that assessment and evaluation cover the four areas of science and scholarship, clinical practice, health and society, professionalism. (B 3.1.2)

- use a reasonable and diverse assessment and evaluation methods depending on different objectives. (B 3.1.3)

- use a system for appeal of assessment and evaluation results. (B 3.1.4)

Quality development standards:

The medical school **should**

- establish assessment and evaluation systems and methods that are compatible with training objectives and curriculum models. (Q 3.1.1)
- actively initiate research of its assessment and evaluation system and methods, and incorporate new assessment and evaluation methods where appropriate. (Q 3.1.2)
- ensure that assessments and evaluations are open to scrutiny by medical education experts. (Q 3.1.3)

3.2 Relationship between assessment and evaluation and learning

Basic standards:

The medical school **must**

- use assessment and evaluation principles, methods and practices that
  - ensure that the intended educational outcomes are met by the students. (B 3.2.1)
  - promote student learning. (B 3.2.2)
  - provide an appropriate balance of formative

and summative assessments and timely feedback to guide learning. (B 3.2.3)

Quality development standards:

The medical school **should**

- encourage both acquisition of the knowledge base and integrated learning by adjusting the number and type of assessment and evaluation of curricular elements. (Q 3.2.1)

- ensure timely, targeted and constructive feedback to students on the basis of assessment and evaluation results. (Q 3.2.2)

Annotations:

- *Assessment and evaluation principles, methods and practices* would design overall correspond to the education objectives, and encourage the use of special types of examinations, e.g. objective structured clinical examination (OSCE), mini clinical evaluation exercise (mini-CEX), direct observation of procedural skills (DOPS), computer-based case simulations (CCS), and the evaluation of entrustable professional activities (EPAs). (A 3.2.1)

- *Summative assessment* is performed after the educational activities, which is used to determine whether the education objectives have been achieved. Summative assessment focuses on the evaluation of performances and learning outcomes. (A 3.2.2)

- *Formative assessment* stresses the combination of education and evaluation procedures, attaches importance to and emphasizes the timely feedback and modification during the course of teaching and learning. Formative assessment is both helpful for the teachers to know their teaching effectiveness and optimize teaching, and for the students to evaluate their own progress in learning and adjust their learning strategies accordingly. (A 3.2.3)

- *Integrated learning* would include consideration of using integrated assessment, while ensuring reasonable tests of knowledge of individual disciplines or subject areas. (A 3.2.4)

3.3 Analysis and feedback of assessment and evaluation results

Basic standards:

The medical school **must**

- analyze the assessment results based on the educational measurement after all the examinations are finished. (B 3.3.1)
- provide feedback on analysis and results of assessment and evaluation to students, faculty and academic affairs administrators. (B 3.3.2)

Quality development standards:

The medical school **should**

- apply the analyzed results in the improvement of teaching and learning. (Q 3.3.1)
- enhance the reform efforts and research of assessments and evaluation. (Q 3.3.2)

Annotation:

- *Analysis of assessment results* includes the degree of difficulties, differentiation, reliability, validity, content coverage, and student performance scores of the tests. (A 3.3.1)

4．Students

4.1   Admission policy and selection

Basic standards:

The medical school **must**

- formulate an admission plan based on the national admission policy and periodically review it for adjustment. (B 4.1.1)

- pay attention to the diversity of students on the premise of guaranteeing the quality of enrolled students. (B 4.1.2)

- have no discrimination and bias under the condition of meeting the requirements of the program. (B 4.1.3)

- make the admission policies and the related information known to the public. (B 4.1.4)

- have a policy and implement a practice for transfer of students from other programs and institutions. (B 4.1.5)

- use a system for appeal of admission decisions. (B 4.1.6)

Quality development standard:

The medical school **should**

- state clearly the relationship between student selection and the mission of the school, the educational program and the graduate outcomes of basic medical education. (Q 4.1.1)

Annotation:

- *Admission policies and the related information* include the school prospectus, programs, admission plan, tuition and fees, scholarships, and mechanism for appeal, etc., and describe the process of student selection and make the curriculum known to the applicants on the internet. (A 4.1.1)

4.2   Student intake

Basic standard:

The medical school **must**

- define the size of student intake based on relevant national policies, the health needs of the community and society, and the educational resources of the school. (B 4.2.1)

Quality development standards:

The medical school **should**

- take the advice of stakeholders into consideration when reviewing and adjusting the size of student intake. (Q 4.2.1)
- make the students intake reflect the orientation of the school and needs of the society. (Q 4.2.2)

Annotations:

- *The health needs of the community and society* would include consideration of national and regional demands for medical workforce as well as gender, ethnicity and other social requirements (socio-cultural and linguistic characteristics of the population), including the potential need of a special recruitment, admission and induction policy for students in remote areas and minorities. (A 4.2.1)
- *Educational resources* would include the consideration of shared use of clinical education resources by the students of other medical specialties. (A 4.2.2)
- *Stakeholders* would include the education and

health authorities, health facilities, faculty and students, and representatives of the public. (A 4.2.3)

4.3 Student counseling and support

Basic standards:

The medical school **must**

- have a system for academic counseling and support of its students. (B 4.3.1)
- offer support and guidance to students in their activities of learning, living, taking part-time jobs and choosing careers. (B 4.3.2)
- have an effective system of psychological counseling. (B 4.3.3)
- allocate resources for student support and pay attention to the building of student affairs team. (B 4.3.4)
- ensure confidentiality in relation to counseling and support. (B 4.3.5)

Quality development standards:

The medical school **should**

- offer individualized academic guidance and counseling based on the student progress in learning. (Q 4.3.1)

- offer students career planning guidance. (Q 4.3.2)

Annotations:

- *Academic counseling* would include questions related to choice of electives, residency preparation, etc. (A 4.3.1)

- *Student support* would include medical services, career guidance, suitable accommodation for students (including disabled students), and implementation of a student aid system offering scholarships, loans, subsidies and allowances for disadvantaged students in need of financial assistance. (A 4.3.2)

- *Individualized academic guidance and counseling* in addition to learning guidance would include appointing academic mentors for individual students or small groups of students. (A 4.3.3)

4.4　Student representative

Basic standards:

The medical school **must**

- formulate and implement a policy, that ensures the participation of student representatives and appropriate participation in the design, management and evaluation of the curriculum, and in other matters relevant to students. (B 4.4.1)

- support students to establish student organizations allowed by law, guide and encourage organized student activities in providing equipment, spaces, and technical and financial support. (B 4.4.2)

Quality development standard:

The medical school **should**

- have student representatives serving in relevant committees, bodies and departments of the school and ensure that they have certain roles to play. (Q 4.4.1)

Annotation:

- *Student organizations* would include relevant bodies for student self-governance, self-education and self-service. (A 4.4.1)

5．Academic Staff/Faculty

5.1 Recruitment and selection policy

Basic standards:

The medical school **must**

- formulate and implement a staff qualification certification and selection system, to make sure that the teachers meet the performance demands in teaching, research and service functions. (B 5.1.1)

- have a well-structured faculty team composed of a sufficient number of qualified academic staff/faculty based on the school mission, scale and instructional model, especially ensure that a sufficient number of full-time teachers with medical background teach basic biomedical sciences related content. (B 5.1.2)

- outline the responsibilities of the academic staff/faculty to ensure an appropriate ratio and balance between teaching, research and service functions. (B 5.1.3)

- set merit criteria for teaching, research and

services, and evaluate the performance of the academic staff/faculty regularly. (B 5.1.4)

- have a corresponding mechanism to ensure that the results of teacher performance evaluation play a role in school decisions for promotions and appointments of academic, administrative or entitlement nature. (B 5.1.5)

- have a corresponding mechanism to ensure that non-medical staff have the necessary knowledge of medicine. (B 5.1.6)

Quality development standards:

The medical school **should**

- in its policy for staff recruitment and selection take into account the school mission and the requirements for reform and development. (Q 5.1.1)

- take into account the reasonable and effective use of personnel expenditure and resources when formulating the selection policy to ensure the balanced development of teaching, research and service functions. (Q 5.1.2)

- have a corresponding mechanism to guarantee

clinical teachers' participation in basic biomedical sciences teaching. (Q 5.1.3)

Annotations:

- *Qualified academic staff/faculty* would indicate that the academic staff/faculty should possess good professional ethics and the scholarship and teaching ability that match their academic ranks, deliver corresponding courses and assume required teaching assignments, and be certified by the corresponding educational authorities. (A 5.1.1)

- *Merits* would be measured by formal qualifications, professional experience, teaching awards, research output, student evaluation and peer recognition. (A 5.1.2)

5.2 Staff activity and staff development

Basic standards:

The medical school **must**

- formulate and effectively implement policies related to faculty training, development, support and appraisal, to ensure that the central focus is on educating students. These policies should

- guarantee the legal rights of the academic staff/faculty. (B 5.2.1)
- recognize and support the professional development of the academic staff/faculty. (B 5.2.2)
- encourage that the academic staff/faculty apply their clinical experience and research findings in teaching. (B 5.2.3)
- ensure that the academic staff/faculty have access to be directly involved in the curriculum design and the decision-making process related to educational management. (B 5.2.4)
- promote the communication among the academic staff/faculty. (B 5.2.5)
- ensure that the academic staff/faculty possess and maintain their competence in teaching, and encourage teaching innovation. (B 5.2.6)
- promote a balance of faculty roles in teaching, research and service functions. (B 5.2.7)

Quality development standards:

The medical school **should**

- have a special institution or department to

formulate development plans for medical staff/faculty and establish long-term training mechanisms. (Q 5.2.1)

- establish a mechanism for the academic staff/faculty to participate in the management and policy-making. (Q 5.2.2)
- have a corresponding policy to ensure a balance of faculty roles in teaching, research and service functions. (Q 5.2.3)
- ensure sufficient knowledge by individual staff members of education objectives and the curriculum. (Q 5.2.4)
- have corresponding mechanisms to ensure mutual communication and cooperation between teachers of different disciplines who undertake teaching tasks, especially basic biomedical teachers and clinical teachers. (Q 5.2.5)

Annotations:

- *Staff activity and development* would involve not only new teachers, but also all the teachers in basic biomedical sciences and clinical sciences. (A 5.2.1)

- *Staff development* would pay attention to the promotion of teaching abilities, and provide training in educational theory, curriculum design, teaching methods and teaching evaluations, as well as consultation, guidance, technical support and feedback. (A 5.2.2)

- *Decision-making process related to educational management* would also include having roles to shape decisions on student admission and services. The school should also ensure that teachers also take part in the decision-making of other important issues. (A 5.2.3)

- *Sufficient knowledge by individual staff members of the curriculum* would include knowledge about overall curriculum content, teaching methods and assessment methods, for the purpose of fostering the cooperation of teachers and integration of curricular contents among different disciplines, and offering students appropriate guidance for learning. (A 5.2.4)

- *Communication among the academic staff/ faculty* would include interdisciplinary and cross-disciplinary communications, and in particular, the communications among teachers of clinical sciences, basic biomedical sciences, public health and preventive medicine sciences and humanities and social sciences. Furthermore, would support staff to attend teaching related academic conferences. (A 5.2.5)

- *Competence in teaching* would include adapting to the educational objectives of the school, following its basic principles, designing appropriate teaching activities, and choosing student assessment methods. (A 5.2.6)

- *A balance of faculty roles in teaching, research and service functions* would include provision of protected time for each function. *Service functions* would include clinical duties in the health care delivery system, student guidance, participation in governance and management and other social services as well. (A 5.2.7)

6. Educational Resources

6.1 Educational funds and allocation of resources

Basic standards:

The medical school **must**

- have reliable and diversified access to fund raising. (B 6.1.1)
- have sufficient financial support to sustain a sound program of medical education and institutional goals. (B 6.1.2)

Quality development standards:

The medical school **should**

- have the autonomy to make overall use of financial and other resources for medical education. (Q 6.1.1)
- support research and implementation of medical education reforms financially. (Q 6.1.2)

Annotations:

- In the *educational founds*, the tuition charged by the medical school must be managed and used according to national regulations. The funds used for teaching and their proportion in the annual final account of the school must meet national regulations. Relevant authorities shall ensure that the funds allocated to medical students meet the needs of medical education. Schools should consider the high cost of medical education when allocating funds used for teaching. (A 6.1.1)

- *Diversified access to fund raising* would include government appropriation, tuitions, investments made by civic organizations and private citizens, donations and funds, supports of affiliated and teaching hospitals, incomes from school-run enterprises and social services, etc. (A 6.1.2)

6.2　Physical facilities

Basic standards:

The medical school **must**

- have sufficient physical facilities for staff and students to ensure that the curriculum can be delivered effectively. (B 6.2.1)
- ensure a learning environment, which is safe for staff, students and patients. (B 6.2.2)
- provide sufficient sites and equipment for simulated clinical training to students. (B 6.2.3)

Quality development standards:

The medical school **should**

- improve the learning and living environment by regularly updating and modifying or extending the physical facilities to match the developments of medical education. (Q 6.2.1)
- update and effectively utilize simulated clinical training equipment to develop simulation-based clinical pedagogies. (Q 6.2.2)

Annotations:

- *Physical facilities* would include all types of class-rooms, multimedia equipment, tutorial rooms, laboratories, equipment, specimen and consumable material for basic medical sciences, clinical skills center and simulation equipment, clinical demonstration rooms, libraries, information technology, network resources and amenities including accommodation and recreational facilities. The physical facilities should consider the humane care for human specimens and animals used for teaching and scientific research. (A 6.2.1)

- *A safe learning environment* refers to the safe learning space provided by the school in the process of teaching, which should ensure the personal and property safety of staff and students; it would provide provisions of necessary information and protection from harmful substances, specimens, organisms, plants and animals, laboratory safety regulations and safety equipment, and publish its policies and procedures for addressing emergency and disaster preparedness. Necessary explanations and training on laboratory safety, pathogen exposure, handling of dangerous and radioactive substances, etc. shall be provided. (A 6.2.2)

6.3   Clinical training resources

Basic standards:

The medical school **must**

- have tertiary class-A affiliated hospitals that can undertake the whole process of clinical teaching, clerkship and internship as clinical teaching sites. (B 6.3.1)
- have sufficient clinical teaching sites to ensure

adequate clinical experience and necessary resources in clinical teaching, including sufficient patients and clinical training facilities. The number of students in the medical specialties and the number of patient beds in these hospitals should have a ratio of less than 1 : 1. (B 6.3.2)

- have enough staff from appropriate disciplines, and with the necessary skills and experience to deliver teaching and support students' learning. (B 6.3.3)

Quality development standard:

The medical school **should**

- continuously evaluate, adapt and improve clinical training resources to meet the needs of teaching and healthcare services. (Q 6.3.1)

Annotations:

- *Affiliated hospitals* are subsidiaries of the medical school, which are under the direct control of the medical school. The school has the right to appoint or dismiss the main responsible person of the affiliated hospital or the affiliated hospital' s organization relationship of the

Communist Party of China belongs to the school. (A 6.3.1)

- *Clinical teaching sites* encompass teaching hospitals, training hospitals and community health centers in addition to the affiliated hospitals. Teaching hospitals, training hospitals, etc. have no affiliation with the medical school. A teaching hospital must meet the following requirements: governmental documents certifying it as a clinical teaching site of a medical school; written agreements between the medical school and the hospital; be capable of and responsible for delivering the medical courses such as clinical teaching, clerkship and internship. A clinical teaching site must have specialized organizations and staff in charge of the administration and management of clinical trainings. (A 6.3.2)

- *Clinical teaching resources* also include adequate numbers of patients with wide range of diseases, in addition to pedagogical equipment. (A 6.3.3)

- *Medical specialties* in this document refer to the medical specialties that award the degree of Bachelor of Medicine, including clinical medicine, anesthesiology, medical radiology, ophthalmology and optometry, psychiatry, radioactive medicine, pediatrics, stomatology, traditional Chinese medicine, clinical discipline of Chinese and western integrative medicine, basic medicine, forensic medicine and preventive medicine, etc. The students of medical specialties include undergraduate students from the above specialties, overseas students taught in Chinese/ English and junior college students. (A 6.3.4)

- *Patient beds* refer to the total in affiliated hospitals and teaching hospitals. The patient beds in affiliated hospital refer to the sum of them in the affiliated comprehensive hospitals and specialized hospitals responsible for clinical teaching and practices. The patient beds in teaching hospitals refer to the number of beds in the teaching hospitals responsible for the whole process of clinical teaching, clerkship and internship and the hospitals should also possess graduate students of clinical medicine, but the patient beds in the specialized hospitals are excluded. The number of patient beds is recognized as the number in the official reports of the hospital submitted to the health authorities at the end of the previous year. The number of patient beds should be the smaller one of the number registered and the number used. (A 6.3.5)

- *Staff* include residents and above, as well as community doctors who meet the teaching requirements of the school. Medical schools need to have access mechanisms for clinical teachers to ensure that they are competent for teaching. (A 6.3.6)

- *Evaluation of clinical training resources* would include the assessment in regards of settings, equipment, number and categories of patients, as well as health practices, supervision and administration to measure whether they meet the teaching requirements. The resources in the affiliated and teaching hospitals shared by students from other medical schools should also be considered. (A 6.3.7)

6.4   Information technology

Basic standards:

The medical school **must**

- own adequate information and communication technology infrastructure and support systems. (B 6.4.1)
- formulate and implement policies which address the effective use of information and communication technology and resources in medical education to ensure the delivery of the educational program. (B 6.4.2)

Quality development standards:

The medical school **should**

- enable teachers and students to use existing and explore appropriate new information technology to support self-directed learning. (Q 6.4.1)
- optimise student access to relevant patient medical record data and health care information systems on the premise of conforming to medical ethics. (Q 6.4.2)
- present and defend virtual learning methods (digital, distance, distributed, or e-learning) as

an alternative or complementary educational approach under appropriate circumstances, including societal emergencies. (Q 6.4.3)

Annotations:

- *Effective use of information and communication technology* would include the use of computers, internal and external networks and other means. This would include coordination with library resources and IT services of the institution. The policy would include common access to all educational items through a learning management system. Information and communication technology would be useful for fostering of students' ability for self-directed learning and life-long learning, and preparing students through continuing professional development (CPD)/ continuing medical education (CME). (A 6.4.1)

- *Distributed learning* means that a varied and planned course of study, designed and developed to address the curriculum for students who are in different locations away from the central teaching institution, supported by teaching and supervisory staff who are also physically or virtually distributed across those locations. Distributed and distance learning is a whole-systems approach, including all teaching and learning, formative and summative assessments, feedback on learning, support for students and teachers, management, and quality assurance. Distributed and distance learning might refer to an entire course, or a part of it. (A 6.4.2)

6.5 Educational expertise

Basic standard:

The medical school **must**

- formulate and implement a policy that has access to educational expertise involved in deciding on important issues concerning medical education, including the development of curriculum, the selection, adjustment and reform of teaching and assessment methods. (B 6.5.1)

Quality development standards:

The medical school **should**

- allow the educational expertise to play an

important role in faculty development. (Q 6.5.1)

- pay attention to the development of on-campus expertise in program evaluations and in research on medical education. (Q 6.5.2)

Annotation:

- *Educational expertise* would rely on experts who have experience in studying and solving problems in medical education and these experts would include teachers, medical doctors, administrators and researchers with research experience in medical education. It can be provided by the school itself or be acquired from another institution. (A 6.5.1)

6.6　Educational exchanges

Basic standards:

The medical school **must**

- formulate and implement a policy for national and international collaboration with other educational institutions. (B 6.6.1)
- facilitate regional and international exchange of staff and students by providing appropriate resources. (B 6.6.2)

- formulate and implement a policy for transfer of educational credits. (B 6.6.3)

Quality development standard:

The medical school **should**

- ensure that exchange is purposefully organized, taking into account the needs of staff and students, respecting the customs of each teaching site and following ethical principles. (Q 6.6.1)

Annotation:

- *A policy for transfer of educational credits* would be facilitated by establishing agreements on mutual recognition of educational elements and through active program coordination between medical schools. It would also be facilitated with the use of a transparent system of credit units and flexible interpretation of course requirements. (A 6.6.1)

7. Program Evaluation

7.1　Mechanisms for program monitoring and evaluation

Basic standards:

The medical school **must**

- have full-time staff for program monitoring and evaluation and establish a mechanism with emphasis on the monitoring and evaluation of curriculum, educational process and outcome. (B 7.1.1)

- establish detailed requirements for all educational components according to the quality standards of medical specialties. (B 7.1.2)

- ensure the relevant results of evaluation improve the curriculum. (B 7.1.3)

- enable the faculty, students and administrators to understand the system of education program monitoring and evaluation. (B 7.1.4)

Quality development standards:

The medical school **should**

- conduct a comprehensive evaluation of the

curriculum regularly and form periodic reports. (Q 7.1.1)

- follow up student progress, such as learning processes, changes in learning abilities, and student life and academic assistance, and give timely feedback to the stakeholders such as students, staff and administrative departments. (Q 7.1.2)

- establish a specialized department for educational evaluation and effectively play its role. (Q 7.1.3)

- provide training for relevant personnel in charge of the evaluation, so that they are able to choose and use appropriate and effective evaluation methods. (Q 7.1.4)

Annotations:

- *Program evaluation* is the process of systematic gathering of information to judge the effectiveness and adequacy of curriculum, educational process and outcomes, so as to provide references for the improvement of education quality and making decisions on education issues. It would imply the use of reliable and valid methods of data collection and analysis. The information and data may include policies, rules and regulations, meeting minutes, joint agreements with other educational institutions; it may also include quality report on undergraduate medical education, evaluation data and results of students, faculties, supervisors, external experts, employers, authorities and other stakeholders on teaching and learning. (A 7.1.1)

- *Program monitoring* would imply the observation and supervision of key aspects of the curriculum, including routine collection of data and so on, which for the purpose of ensuring that the educational process is on track and for identifying any areas in need of intervention. Such information collection is often a part of the administrative process related to enrollment, student assessment, graduation, etc. (A 7.1.2)

- *Periodic reports* addressing the context of the educational process, the specific components of the curriculum, the educational outcomes acquired, and its social accountability. The context of the educational process would include the institutional environment, resource environment, learning environment and culture of the medical school. The educational outcomes can be reflected through the examinations organized inside and outside the school [such as comprehensive examinations at different phases, the Level Test of Basic Medical Education (undergraduate) in Medical Schools, the National Medical Licensing Examination (NMLE), qualifying examinations for standardized residency training, etc.], career choices, employment destinations, and performance of graduates, which can be used as a reference for the improvement of undergraduate medical education. (A 7.1.3)

7.2   Teacher and student feedback

Basic standard:

The medical school **must**

- apply multiple evaluation methods, systematically seek and analyse information, and give feedback to teachers and students. (B 7.2.1)

Quality development standard:

The medical school **should**

- use feedback results for curriculum development and achieve expected improvement. (Q 7.2.1)

Annotation:

- *Feedback* would include information about the processes and outcomes of the educational programs. It would also include information about school policies and regulations, malpractices or inappropriate conducts involving teachers or students with or without legal consequences. (A 7.2.1)

7.3   Performance of students and graduates

Basic standard:

The medical school **must**

- analyze performance of cohorts of students and graduates in relation to its mission, intended educational outcomes, curriculum, and provision of resources. (B 7.3.1)

Quality development standard:

The medical school **should**

- use the results of student development evaluations

and graduate analysis to shape admission policies, revise education programs and offer consultation services to students. (Q 7.3.1)

Annotations:

- *Performance of cohorts of students and graduates* can be reflected by collecting and using various education outcomes data, as well as by indicating the degree of completion of education objectives. (A 7.3.1)

- *Student development* includes physical and mental development and academic development of students at school. The measurement and analysis of academic development include learning duration, test scores, test passing rate, academic completion rate and dropout rate. The school can make value-added assessment on students' development through questionnaires, symposiums, academic achievement data analysis, etc. (A 7.3.2)

- Measures of *graduate analysis* would include information about career choice, performance in clinical service delivery and post-graduation promotion as well as other job performance measures for graduates. (A 7.3.3)

7.4 Involvement of stakeholders

Basic standard:

The medical school **must**

- in its program monitoring and evaluation activities involve its principal stakeholders on campus such as academic staff, students and administrators. (B 7.4.1)

Quality development standard:

The medical school **should**

- encourage other stakeholders to contribute to its course and program evaluation and have access to the evaluation results. (Q 7.4.1)
- seek other stakeholders' feedback on the performance of graduates and on the curriculum. (Q 7.4.2)

Annotation:

- *Other stakeholders* would include other representatives of academic and administrative staff, representatives of the community and public (e.g., users of the health care system), education and health care authorities, professional organizations, medical scientific bodies and postgraduate educators. (A 7.4.1)

8. Scientific Research

8.1 Education and scientific research

Basic standards:

The medical school **must**

- formulate and implement a policy that promotes the coordinated development of scientific research and education programs. (B 8.1.1)
- strengthen the study of medical education and management, to provide theoretical basis for the educational reform and development. (B 8.1.2)

Quality development standards:

The medical school **should**

- incorporate scientific research activities and outcomes into the educational process, to train students' ability in scientific methods, scientific thinking and spirits of science, and to ensure positive interactions of scientific research and education activities. (Q 8.1.1)

- establish special medical education research department to play a practical role in promoting medical education reform and improving teachers' educational scientific research ability. (Q 8.1.2)

Annotation:

- *Medical education research* refers to the educational scientific research carried out according to relevant theories on medical education activities, mainly focusing on the theoretical, practical, and social aspects of medical education. The purpose is to deeply reveal the laws of medical education and provide theoretical and research support for medical education reform. (A 8.1.1)

8.2　Scientific research by staff

Basic standards:

The medical school **must**

- encourage academic staff to conduct scientific research and provide basic resources needed for the complementary development of scientific research and education. (B 8.2.1)
- ensure academic staff to be equipped with

corresponding ability in scientific research. (B 8.2.2)

Quality development standard:

The medical school **should**

- have the corresponding mechanisms to guarantee involvement of academic staff in the research of medical education, so as to enhance the teaching effectiveness. (Q 8.2.1)

8.3   Scientific research of students

Basic standards:

The medical school **must**

- use the scientific research activities as an important pathway to foster students' scientific literacy and creativity, and adopt effective measures to provide students with opportunities and resources needed for scientific research. (B 8.3.1)

- actively engage in activities which are instrumental in fostering students' research competencies, such as incorporating comprehensive experiments and self-designed experiments in the curriculum, holding academic lectures and organizing scientific research teams. (B 8.3.2)

- make students understand the basic methods and ethical principles of medical science research. (B 8.3.3)

Quality development standard:

The medical school **should**

- provide funds for the scientific research activities of students. (Q 8.3.1)

9. Governance and Administration

9.1 Governance system and mechanism

Basic standards:

The medical school **must**

- articulate its governance system and structures among the university, medical school and affiliated hospitals, define the management functions of the three, and establish an effective management mechanism among university, medical school and affiliated hospitals, so as to ensure the integrity of medical education, as well as the effective operation and sustainable development of teaching. (B 9.1.1)

- establish functional committees in its governance structures to review and discuss important issues involving the curriculum, educational reform and scientific research. The committees should include principal stakeholders on campus such as the school leaders, representatives of teachers and students, and administrative staff. (B 9.1.2)

Quality development standards:

The medical school **should**

- in its corresponding committees include other stakeholders such as representatives of governmental authorities and regulatory bodies, health care sectors, and the community and public. (Q 9.1.1)
- ensure transparency of the work of governance and its decisions. (Q 9.1.2)

Annotations:

- *Governance* is primarily concerned with policy making, the processes of establishing general institutional and program policies and also with control of the implementation of the policies. The institutional and program policies would normally encompass decisions on the mission of the medical education, the curriculum, admission policy, staff recruitment and selection policy and decisions on interaction and linkage with medical practice and the health sector as well as other external relations. (A 9.1.1)

- Members of the *committees* should be widely representative. The activities of the committees should be organized by the persons in charge, and recorded in details concerning the time, issues discussed, decisions and participants. (A 9.1.2)

- *Transparency* would be obtained by newsletters, web-information or disclosure of meeting minutes. (A 9.1.3)

9.2　Medical education leadership

Basic standards:

The medical school **must**

- clearly illustrate the management responsibilities and authority in terms of human, financial, and physical resources of its medical education leadership on medical education, and ensure the effective execution accordingly. (B 9.2.1)

- pay attention to the professional background of the leaders in charge of medical education. (B 9.2.2)
- ensure that the medical education leadership is relatively stable. (B 9.2.3)

Quality development standard:

The medical school **should**

- periodically evaluate the performance of its medical education leadership in the process of teaching management. (Q 9.2.1)

Annotation:

- *Medical education leadership* refers to the leaders who are mainly responsible for the medical education and the personnel working in administrative department who are responsible for making decisions on academic matters such as teaching, scientific research and services. (A 9.2.1)

9.3　Administrative staff and management

Basic standards:

The medical school **must**

- have a complete administrative staff team with effective management structures and advanced educational philosophy that is appropriate to support implementation of medical education. (B 9.3.1)

- establish a sound management system and operating procedures to ensure rational deployment of resources. (B 9.3.2)

- have corresponding measures to ensure that the administrative staff understand medical education and the whole process of it. (B 9.3.3)

Quality development standard:

The medical school **should**

- regularly evaluate and improve the management of medical education. (Q 9.3.1)

9.4　Interaction with health sector

Basic standards:

The medical school **must**

- have constructive interaction and communication

with the health related sectors for support to medical education. (B 9.4.1)

- sign agreements with relevant health sectors, so as to ensure the successful delivery of the curricula. (B 9.4.2)

Quality development standard:

The medical school **should**

- formalize extensive cooperation and exchanges with medical and health related sectors, and ensure a sustainable development of the cooperation and exchanges. (Q 9.4.1)

Annotations:

- *Relevant health sectors* would not only include the healthcare delivery system, whether public or private, medical research institutions, but the institutions and regulatory bodies with implications for health promotion and disease prevention, etc. (A 9.4.1)
- To *formalize extensive cooperation and exchanges* would mean entering into formal agreements, stating the content and forms of collaboration, and/or establishing joint projects. (A 9.4.2)

10．Reform and Development

Basic standards:

The medical school **must**

- systematically design the reform of medical education, carry out evidence-based research, and scientifically evaluate the effect of the reform. (B 10.0.1)

- establish corresponding mechanism, regularly review and evaluate self-development, understand its own problems and make continuous improvement. (B 10.0.2)

Quality development standards:

The medical school **should**

- base the process of continuous development on prospective studies and analyses and on results of local evaluation and the literature on medical education. (Q 10.0.1)

- ensure that the process of continuous development and restructuring leads to the revision of its policies and practices in accordance with past experience, present activities and future perspectives. (Q 10.0.2)

- adjust education strategies based on changes in health needs and social and technological development trends. (Q 10.0.3)